Reversing Type 2 Diabetes

Foreword by Mike Adams

Written by Vicki Batts

First Edition, First Printing

Foreword by Mike Adams
Written by Vicki Batts
Edited by Natural News Editors

Disclaimer: This book is offered for information purposes only and is protected under freedom of speech. It is not medical advice nor should it be construed as such. Nothing in this book is intended to diagnose or treat any disease. Always work with a qualified health professional before making any changes to your diet, prescription drug use, lifestyle or exercise activities. This information is provided as-is, and the reader assumes all risks from the use, non-use or misuse of this information.

Table of Contents

Foreword by Mike Adams

I have great news to share with all those who are diabetic: diabetes has a cause. That very cause means that there is something you can do for your condition. By understanding the disease and what causes it, you can change the results you see in your own body. Even in many advanced cases, diabetes can be reversed at least partially, with reduced dependence on insulin and diabetes drugs.

For those who haven't yet been diagnosed with diabetes but may have been told they have pre-diabetes, or even hypoglycemia, the good news here is that you can prevent diabetes and make sure it never gets expressed in your body. This book explains the fundamentals that the medical industry refuses to teach. In these pages, you will find information that your doctor doesn't know because it wasn't taught in medical school, and that the drug companies hope and pray you never learn, because the minute you learn this information you are no longer a highly-profitable, lifelong customer of the medical system's "disease management racket."

Diabetes is not something the medical establishment is interested in preventing, reversing, or curing. That's because managing diabetes is so incredibly profitable and it generates a recurring revenue stream because the underlying causes of diabetes are never addressed. As long as the disease is never reversed, the patient remains dependent on doctors, pharmaceuticals, and insulin, all of which generate enormous revenues for the drug industry and the hospitalization sector of our economy.

The drug companies are counting on your diabetes to generate repeat revenues for them, so they neglect to teach people how to prevent this disease using simple, completely natural principles founded in good science, biochemical cause and effect, and compassion for human beings.

You see, as a lab science director at CWCLabs.com, and as the editor of NaturalNews.com, I've spent over 14 years teaching people how to heal themselves without destroying their health through toxic medical intervention such as pharmaceuticals, chemotherapy, and surgery. I've interviewed diabetics, and I've met people who have reversed type 2 diabetes in as little as four days simply by changing what they eat.

Nearly every case of diabetes that I've ever seen is reversible. It simply requires the knowledge of knowing what causes diabetes versus what allows your body to heal itself and reverse diabetes. To get there, you first have to understand that diabetes is not an infection, it's not a parasite, and it isn't an epidemic. You weren't struck by diabetes in the same way that you can catch malaria, for example.

Diabetes is simply a name, a medical label, given to a set of medical symptoms that are observations of your body's expression of biochemistry. When that expression gets out of balance, it's called disease. When that expression is restored back into balance, it's called health.

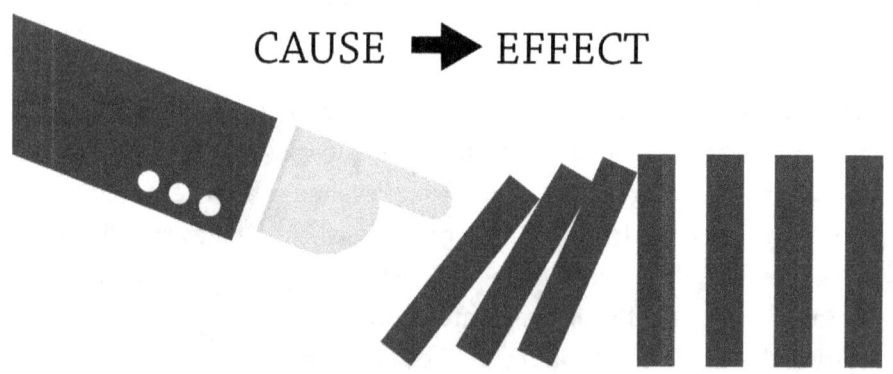

CAUSE ➡ EFFECT

If you don't believe in cause & effect, eat anything you want
(and suffer the consequences).

You alone have the full power to change your body's expression of health versus disease by changing the inputs that you provide to your body. What are these inputs? They obviously include things like food, but also they can also include nutritional supplements, pharmaceuticals, environmental chemicals, personal care products, the water that you drink, the sunlight that you get, the air that you're breathing, and so on. All of these things are inputs.

Physical exertion and exercise is also another form of input. Quality of sleep and mindset are additional inputs. All of these things affect the health outcome that you experience. If you are currently experiencing a health outcome that is labeled 'disease', then you'll be happy to know that you can change that outcome by changing the inputs that affect your body.

That's what this book is primarily about. Here, you'll learn that diabetes does not have to be a passive disease. Disease progression doesn't have to be something that happens outside of your control. Type 2 diabetes, in particular, is something that has a root cause. When that root cause is avoided or altered, then you get different results; a healing in the body that can restore balance and physiological health to the point where you may no longer even be labeled "diabetic." Achieving that is simpler than you think, but it does require you to make changes in your lifestyle choices.

If you are currently a type 2 diabetic, there's little question that you got there through a combination of a lack of physical exercise combined with very high intake of nutrient-depleted processed foods, such as sodas, white flour, white sugar, and other factory foods. These foods are devoid of real nutrition, but they're very high in empty calories. When combined with a sedentary lifestyle – a lack of exercise – they alter your body's sensitivity to insulin, and they lead to an expression of physiological conditions that get diagnosed as type 2 diabetes.

The drug industry wants you to control these symptoms using toxic pharmaceuticals, some of which cause liver damage. But you have options that are far safer, less costly, and can be permanent. You have the option of eliminating all of the toxic processed foods from your life and bringing in high-potency, nutrient-dense super foods that contain the healing minerals and phytonutrients, which are plant-based nutrients, that can help your body heal and recover and rebalance itself so that you are no longer qualified as diabetic. There's a certain level of physical activity that must go along with this as well, but it can be accomplished with something as simple as walking or swimming or even slowly and steadily climbing flights of stairs as a form of exercise.

Making these changes is simpler than most people might suspect, and these changes can free you from a lifetime of dependence on toxic drugs, and doctors, and hospitals, and possibly even amputations if diabetes progresses in your body.

It's interesting to note that the medical industry hopes you never have access to this knowledge. This knowledge is empowering. It teaches people like yourself how to heal yourself so that you don't need the toxic, high-cost medical interventions offered by the for-profit medical system. By learning the information in this book, you can become a freer and more healthful individual who has more options in your life. And instead of sending money to the drug companies and doctors on a regular basis to "manage" your disease, you can reinvest that money in your own joys or, perhaps, in support of family members, because you no longer have that disease.

Within these pages you'll find the recipe, if you will, for unlocking this inner healing potential that you were born with. You'll learn how to reverse and prevent type 2 diabetes, and how to live the rest of your life as a healthy, self-empowered individual who is expressing the inner biochemical balance that your body was meant to express.

You do not have to be a victim for life, but you do have to make determined changes. If you keep doing the things that you've done so far, which developed diabetes, then, obviously, you're not going to get any different results. In other words - if you want different results, you need to engage in different inputs. Fortunately, those inputs are very easy to describe, and that's what you'll learn in this book.

Finally, I do strongly recommend that you work with a qualified naturopathic physician to help guide you along this journey. If you begin to make these changes and you are currently on insulin, you may need to reduce insulin, and eventually eliminate it, with the help of a qualified health professional. Your need for insulin may diminish quite rapidly as you begin to change your diet and level of exercise.

There are many people who used to be dependent on insulin who are now completely free from it simply by changing what they eat, how they nourish their bodies, and what level of physical activity they choose to pursue. But this needs to be done carefully, under the guidance of someone who's qualified as a holistic physician and who understands all the realms of nutrition, pharmaceuticals, exercise physiology and the body's healing process. So, even as you learn the information in this book, find a qualified complementary or alternative medicine naturopathic physician who can help you achieve the goal of being completely diabetes-free for the rest of your life.

For nearly everyone who might read this book, that goal is achievable, but it doesn't happen automatically. It requires effort on your part and it does require avoiding the things that cause diabetes. So be prepared to make some changes, but also feel empowered in the fact that those changes can set you free from the prison of medical dependence and pharmaceutical intervention - if you allow yourself to continue down that road, it will probably cause far more problems for you in the end.

When people are type 2 diabetic, if they don't reverse that condition they will eventually end up with heart disease or cancer or other complications stemming from the diabetes. So think of this journey as not just preventing or reversing one disease, but as a larger journey of discovery to save your own life in many different ways. This is about empowering you to save yourself and thereby prevent yourself from becoming another money-making victim of the pharmaceutical industry, the junk food industry, and all the other corporate entities that prey upon death and disease to enhance and fatten their bottom lines.

You have the power to deconstruct your disease and rebuild your health — you just need to use the right tools.

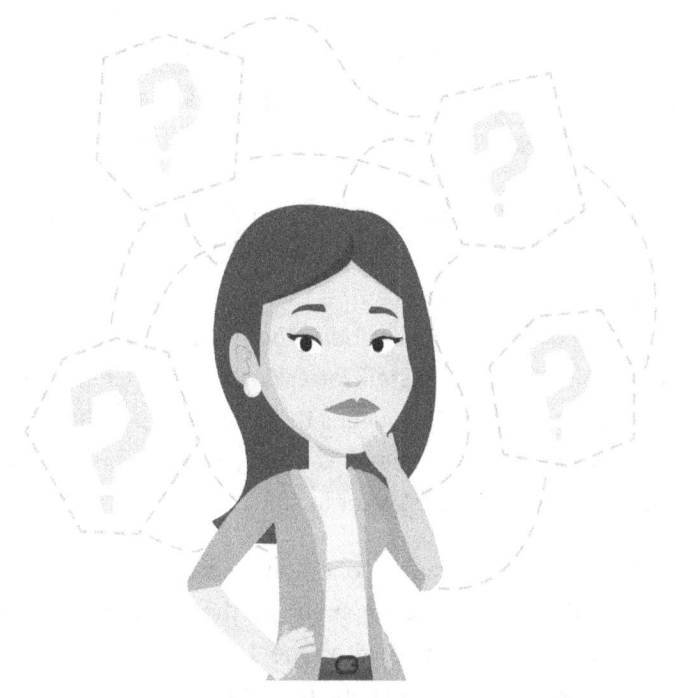

Chapter 1 – What is Type 2 Diabetes?

To begin deconstructing diabetes, we must first build an understanding of the condition. Type 2 diabetes is the most common form of diabetes mellitus. It's often considered a lifelong, chronic illness that is characterized by high blood sugar levels.[1] In normal, healthy individuals, plenty of insulin is produced by beta cells in the pancreas. Insulin is a hormone that stimulates cells to absorb and store sugar, or glucose, from the bloodstream.

In type 2 diabetes, however, the body has developed insulin resistance and no longer responds to the hormone effectively, or a person's pancreas is no longer capable of producing enough insulin for their body. This results in hyperglycemia, or high blood sugar. The best way to manage the condition is by maintaining a healthy weight, losing weight if you are overweight and by following a healthy diet.[2]

Type 2 diabetes is also associated with severe complications such as neuropathy (nerve damage), heart disease, coronary artery disease, atherosclerosis, kidney damage that can lead to end-stage renal disease and many other damaging conditions.[3]

Type 2 diabetes differs from type 1 diabetes in that it is not an autoimmune condition. Type 2 diabetics can, and do, make their own insulin. Through diet and exercise, the condition can be managed without medication and can be reversed with enough dedication. The main characteristic of type 1 diabetes is that the immune system attacks the body's beta cells, which form insulin in the pancreas. This means that the body produces little or no insulin for circulation. Type 1 diabetes is usually evident early in childhood, but it is possible to develop type 1 later in life.

Type 1 diabetes is an autoimmune condition, and while making good food choices is imperative to the management of the condition, it cannot be cured through food alone. People with type 1 diabetes cannot make their own insulin and need to have that supplemented with medication – which is why it is sometimes referred to as insulin-dependent diabetes. If you have type 1 diabetes, it is always recommended to follow a healthy diet and be active – along with taking your insulin appropriately.[4]

"Type 3 diabetes" refers to the evidence-based hypothesis that Alzheimer's disease is a variation of diabetes mellitus in which insulin resistance solely affects the brain.[5]

What Is Insulin?

Insulin is a hormone secreted by beta cells located in the pancreas. Plasma glucose levels mainly moderate secretion of insulin. Insulin needs to bind to a cell receptor site in order to perform its biological functions. Once insulin has bound to a receptor, its end result of activation will vary based upon cell-type. The activation of insulin reception may include alterations in metabolism, transcription rates, protein translocation and the growth rate of responsive cells.[6]

In most tissue, such as skeletal muscle and adipose tissue, insulin generates an increase in the uptake of glucose by stimulating an increase in the number of plasma glucose transporters (GLUTs). There are several different types of glucose transporters, often found in different tissues. For example, GLUT4 is found in insulin responsive tissues, such as skeletal muscle and adipose tissue, while GLUT3 is primarily found in neurons. [6]

What Causes the Body to Develop Insulin Resistance?

A variety of genetic and environmental factors have been found to lead to insulin resistance. Genetic predisposition can certainly make a person more likely to develop insulin resistance, but research suggests that genetics is not the only player in the onset of this terrible disease.

Dr. Jeffrey Pessin, from the Department of Physiology and Biophysics at the University of Iowa, wrote in the summary of an article published in *The Journal of Clinical Investigations*, "Finally, it must be considered that there may be no single or common defect that underlies peripheral insulin resistance. Most likely, insulin resistance is really a complex phenomenon in which several genetic defects combine with environmental stresses, such as obesity or infections, to generate the phenotype."[7]

Pessin suggests that there may be no single cause to insulin resistance and that its cause may indeed be the perfect storm of circumstance. Given what is already known about the risk factors to developing insulin resistance – such as a poor diet, being overweight and a life of inactivity – it seems logical to entertain the idea that perhaps there is more than just one direct cause.

Most people with type 2 diabetes are overweight or obese. This creates a two-prong effect. Being overweight makes it more difficult for your pancreas to produce enough insulin and it makes it more difficult to utilize the insulin that is produced efficiently.[2] Obesity has long been associated with the type of systemic inflammation related to the development of diabetes.[6]

How Insulin Works:

- Secreted by beta cells in pancreas
- After entering blood stream, insulin binds to a receptor
- These receptors for insulin are located in bodily tissues
- Once insulin binds to a receptor, it can exact its effects
- In most tissues, insulin increases the absorption of glucose
- Insulin triggers release of glucose transporters, which pro motes glucose absorption
- Different types of tissue may have different types of glucose transporters

There is also evidence that suggests the accumulation of cellular ceramides may be associated with the onset of diabetes. Ceramide synthesis has been shown to be induced by many things, such as inflammation, chemothera- peutics and excessive saturated fatty acid intake. Ceramides' capacity to block insulin receptor signals lies in their ability to block the receptors from activating the downstream effector, kinase.

Experiments on both skeletal muscle cells and adipocytes (fat cells) have shown that ceramides hinder the insulin-stimulated uptake of glucose, blocking the translocation of GLUT4 (a glucose transporter) to the plasma membrane, as well as impeding the synthesis of glycogen. This evidence suggests that ceramides have the potential to induce insulin resistance through this obstruction of kinase activation.[6]

Recently, Sir Muir Gray announced that he believed that type 2 diabetes should be renamed to "Walking Deficiency Syndrome" due to his finding that lifestyle factors play a substantial role in the onset of the condition. Sir Muir feels that diabetes is not a disease in the true sense of the term, and that our modern inactive lives are the real culprit behind the development of insulin resistance and type 2 diabetes.[8]

Sir Muir has worked for the UK's NHS since 1972 and is an honorary professor at Oxford University. According to him, moving around more and spending less time on the sofa is one of the most helpful things a person can do for their health. And he has a point: the condition is largely preventable, especially with modifications to diet and lifestyle. Sir Muir maintains that this "disease" is a product of modern environment, and that the cause of insulin resistance lies solely at the feet of the inactive individual.[8] To put it simply, his research suggests that the biological effects of inactivity and other aspects of modern life are what cause this condition to develop.

There are also many nutritional aspects to diabetes. Certain foods or ingredients may cause diabetes, while others are thought to help heal it. At a micronutrient level, there are many nutrient deficiencies that can also contribute to the onset of type 2 diabetes. Chapter 4 will cover all the nutritional aspects of diabetes in-depth.

Risk Factors for the Onset of Type 2 Diabetes

Excess weight is one of the most common risk factors for the onset of insulin resistance and, consequently, type 2 diabetes. Belly fat in particular is believed to be one of the key factors in the development of chronic illness and inflammation. Though once perceived as merely energy storage, newer research shows that may not be the case. Research suggests that fat cells produce hormones that can cause serious health issues such as cardiovascular disease and high blood pressure in addition to insulin resistance.[9]

Physical inactivity is another co-conspirator in the development of type 2 diabetes. Besides the fact that a sedentary lifestyle predisposes you to the risk factor of obesity, being inactive reduces your insulin sensitivity. Muscle is one of the primary storage facilities for glucose, and being physically active allows your muscles to use up their glucose stores and receive new glucose from the bloodstream.

Studies show that muscles are more sensitive to insulin after exercise, increasing insulin absorption from the blood, reversing insulin resistance and lowering blood sugar levels.[9]

Controllable Risk Factors for Type 2 Diabetes:

- Sedentary lifestyle and lack of physical activity
- Poor dietary habits
- Low intake of vitamin D and fiber
- High intake of added sugars and fats
- Being overweight or obese
- Smoking

Diet is also a burgeoning factor in the rise of type 2 diabetes and, with ongoing research – more dietary factors continue to be found. One key dietary factor is vitamin D. One study performed by Dr. Esther Krug, endocrinologist at Sinai Hospital in Baltimore and assistant professor of medicine at the Johns Hopkins University School of Medicine, and her colleagues, found that 91% of 124 surveyed type 2 diabetic patients had vitamin D deficiency or insufficient levels of vitamin D. This astounding prevalence of deficiency and their other findings strongly suggest that vitamin D levels are inversely related to the onset of type 2 diabetes.[10]

In addition to low dietary intakes of vitamin D, low-fiber, high-sugar diets are also commonly associated with the onset of type 2 diabetes. These types of foods are associated with more rapid absorption into the bloodstream, resulting in blood sugar and insulin spikes, and are often referred to as "high-glycemic foods." Replacing high-glycemic foods with low-glycemic foods, such as whole grains, has been shown to reduce the risk of developing type 2 diabetes and improve glucose control in people who already have diabetes.[11]

Excessive intake of dietary fats, particularly saturated fatty acids, is also associated with the development of cellular stress, particularly on the endoplasmic reticula and mitochondria. An increase of mitochondrial fat oxidation can lead to the production of reactive oxygen species, which are known to lead to insulin resistance. Excess fatty acid intake has also been shown to interfere with normal insulin receptor mediated signal transduction, also leading to insulin resistance. A high intake of saturated fatty acids is also shown to increase the accumulation of cellular ceramides, which can also impede insulin receptor signaling. Excessive intakes of saturated fatty acids may also reduce insulin secretion from the pancreas.[6]

Another risk factor in the onset of type 2 diabetes is smoking cigarettes. Cigarettes raise blood sugar levels and lead to insulin resistance. Smoking more than 20 cigarettes, or more than one pack, per day nearly doubles a person's likelihood of developing type 2 diabetes in comparison to non-smokers.[12]

There are also some risks for type 2 diabetes that cannot be controlled. Individuals whose parents or siblings have type 2 diabetes are more likely to develop it themselves. Age can also play a role, as people over the age of 45 are especially prone to developing type 2 diabetes. Race is also understood to be a risk factor. African Americans, Asian Americans, Hispanic Americans and Native Americans are all more likely to develop type 2 diabetes than Caucasians. It is not entirely understood at this time why being of a certain race may predispose a person to be more likely to develop this condition.[13] People in these risk groups should be aware of their heightened vulnerability towards this disease.

The Complications of Diabetes

Type 2 diabetes may seem inconsequential from the outside, but it most assuredly is not. Some of the most common complications in diabetes include heart and cardiovascular disease, kidney damage, nerve damage, foot damage, skin conditions and Alzheimer's disease. These complications are extremely serious, and many of them can lead to life-threatening circumstances if not managed properly.

It is also important to note that uncontrolled blood glucose increases the risks for the development of many of these conditions and often the severity in which these conditions are experienced. Conversely, properly managed and maintained blood glucose levels are associated with a reduction in diabetic complication risks.[13]

Diabetic heart disease is caused by the excess glucose in the bloodstream. Many people don't realize this, but the excessive glucose molecules in their bloodstream can lead to the development of plaques along their arterial walls, leading to atherosclerosis, or hardening of the arteries. As the plaque continues to thicken, the artery narrows – reducing the amount of blood that can flow freely to your heart. Over time, a section of plaque may tear open. Blood cell fragments called platelets stick to the injury site as they travel along through the bloodstream.

As the platelets clump together, they inevitably form blood clots. Clots can block your arteries and lead to death. People with type 2 diabetes have higher amounts of these substances that can cause plaques and blood clots.[14]

In addition to raising the risk of heart and cardiovascular disease, kidney damage and disease is another cause for concern in people with type 2 diabetes. In fact, diabetes is the leading cause of kidney failure in the United States. Diabetic kidney disease can take several years to develop. It begins with small amounts of albumin, a blood protein, seeping into the urine. Because kidney filtration is often still functioning normally at this early stage, this symptom can go unnoticed for quite some time.

As it progresses, more albumin leaks into the urine, becoming what is called "proteinuria" or high protein in the urine.[15] High blood sugar levels cause the kidneys to filter too much blood, and over time this damages their delicate filtration system.[15] The severity of kidney damage is gauged by the eGFR, or estimated glomerular filtration rate. This rate is determined by the amount of creatinine in the urine.

Creatinine is a waste product that should normally be filtered out by the kidneys, and as the efficacy of the kidney's filtration system goes down, the level of creatinine in the urine increases. Proper blood glucose management is imperative to the prevention and management of kidney disease for people with type 2 diabetes.[15]

Diabetes was the seventh leading cause of death in the United States in 2014
(Type 1, Type 2 diabetes numbers included)

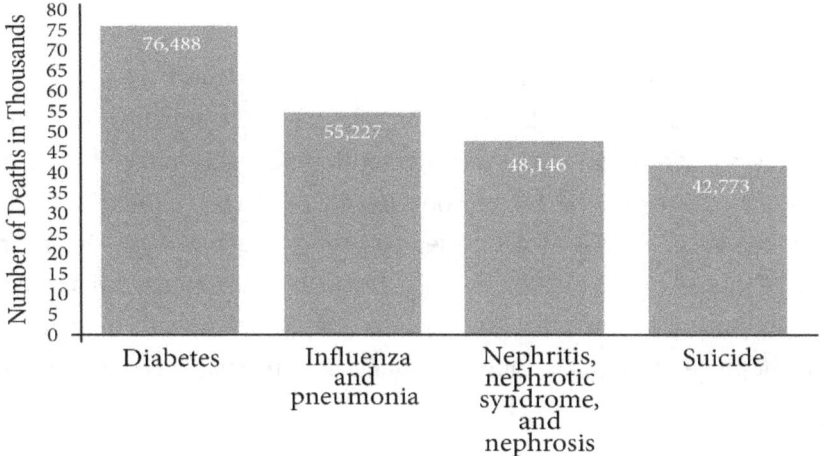

Source: CDC.gov

Nerve damage and foot damage in diabetics is extremely common. Excess blood sugar can cause damage to capillaries – tiny blood vessels – that feed oxygen and nutrients to your nerves. Damage to these blood vessels can lead to the nerves ceasing function. Nerve damage often begins with tingling, numbness, pain or burning sensations at the tips of the fingers or toes and spreads upwards. Continued poor blood glucose control can lead to permanent damage and loss of feeling in the affected limb.

Foot damage and amputation is especially common in the case of diabetic nerve damage. Both damaged nerves and poor blood flow are a direct result of uncontrolled blood sugar and affect the feet with poor wound healing capacity and an increased likelihood that wounds and infections will go unnoticed for long periods of time – which makes toe, foot and leg amputations quite common in diabetics.[13]

Damaged capillaries can occur throughout the body, leading to eye problems and skin conditions. Diabetic retinopathy (damaged capillaries of the retina) can lead to eventual blindness. Type 2 diabetes also increases the risks of developing cataracts and glaucoma as you age. Skin conditions, such as rashes, bacterial infections and fungal infections, are more common in diabetics as well.[13]

In addition to the host of physical ailments and diseases associated with type 2 diabetes, cognitive degeneration disorders are common as well. Brain changes associated with vascular dementia and Alzheimer's disease are common in diabetics. Diabetes is considered a risk factor in the onset of vascular dementia. Damaged capillaries can cause brain damage due to decreased or obstructed blood flow. Mild cognitive impairments are also common in individuals with diabetes as they age. Difficulty with memory and thought processes that are more pronounced than usual is a common symptom of this.

It is hypothesized that the link between these cognitive impairments and diabetes has something to do with the way type 2 diabetes negatively affects the body's capacity to use glucose and respond to insulin.[17] This is especially significant when you consider the fact that the brain is one of the body's primary users of glycogen (synthesized from glucose), and uses about 75% of expended glycogen stores daily. Insulin serves to activate the synthesis of glycogen, as well as inhibit glycogenolysis, or the break down of glycogen for energy.[18] The suggestion that a disease, such as type 2 diabetes, which interferes with the bodily response to insulin and cellular uptake of glucose might cause cognitive defects is not a farfetched one, especially when the brain's considerable expenditure of glycogen is taken into account.

Research has also found that decreasing your chances of diabetes also lowers your risk of developing dementia and other cognitive degenerative conditions.[17]

Diabetes Diagnosis

The main testing modality for type 2 diabetes is a simple A1C, or glycated hemoglobin, test. This blood test looks for the average blood glucose level of the last two to three months. After diagnosis, a person may receive three or four A1C tests per year. After diagnosis, it is up to the individual to make the necessary life style changes to stay healthy. A person may need to check their blood sugar levels daily, change their diet, increase their activity levels, reduce their weight or stop smoking to increase their odds of successfully managing their diabetes.[19]

Type 2 diabetes is a serious condition. The number of life-threatening and debilitating conditions it is associated with is truly astounding. It may be hard to believe that something that seems as simple as your blood sugar levels can have so many ill effects on your body, but it's true. Failure to manage diabetes can leave you with catastrophic complications and a lifetime of hospital bills, or worse.

Perhaps one of the most frightening things about type 2 diabetes is the fact that is has reached epidemic proportions in the United States. According to the CDC, 1.4 million new cases of diabetes were reported in 2014. *New* cases, meaning not including people who were previously diagnosed. In 1980, there were less than half a million new cases for the year. The number of new type 2 diabetes cases nearly tripled in 24 years.[20]

Even more unsettling, a recent study conducted by the Centers for Disease Control with researchers from Emory University in Atlanta found that people with diabetes have lot less to look forward to later in life. The study reviewed health records of 20,008 people over the age of 50 from 1998 to 2012 that had been collected as part of the Health and Retirement Study. On average, diabetics developed a disability seven years earlier than non-diabetics and spent one to two more years in a disabled state than non-diabetics as well. Diabetics died roughly four and a half years earlier than their unaffected counterparts as well.[21]

Worse still, the rates of childhood type 2 diabetes and obesity have begun to skyrocket. 18% of children aged 6–11 and 21% of children aged 12–19 can be categorized as obese. Even being obese or overweight throughout childhood and adolescence carries increased risks for the development of type 2 diabetes later in life, if not in childhood.[22] Obesity is one of the leading factors in the onset of childhood type 2 diabetes. It has also been shown that the progression of obesity-related insulin resistance is much faster in children than adults. Children with a first- or second-degree relative with type 2 diabetes, such as parents, grandparents or siblings, are more likely to develop the condition as well.[23]

Type 2 diabetes may seem like it is just about blood sugar on the surface, but the truth is that is a deeply rooted disease that can negatively impact your body, your life and your family. Nearly 180,000 people are living with kidney failure related to diabetes.[15] Countless others live with horrific complications and disabilities directly related to their diabetes.

The good news is that type 2 diabetes is a highly treatable condition. Unlike type 1 diabetes, type 2 is not an autoimmune condition. Type 2 diabetes can be managed with a healthy diet and lifestyle changes.[4]

For example, studies show that losing just 5–7% of your body weight (if you are overweight) and exercising for just 30 minutes a day can help reduce your chances of developing type 2 diabetes significantly.[6]

Chapter 2 – The Conventional Treatment of Diabetes and Its Shortcomings

Understanding the basics of mainstream diabetes treatment is essential to understanding why it doesn't work. The conventional treatment of type 2 diabetes includes some fairly simple suggestions. The first is to eat a healthier diet. The general idea is to eat more fruits, vegetables and whole grains, and reduce the intake of sweets, animal products and refined carbohydrates. The second suggestion is to be more physically active. This is because physical activity helps lower your blood sugar. The goal is usually about 30 minutes a day, five times a week. Monitoring your blood sugar levels is also recommended. At first, it is suggested to check your blood glucose levels fairly frequently, up to three or four times a day. Once a person gains better control of their blood sugar and achieves consistently balanced glucose levels, the frequency of testing can be reduced. Weight loss is also recommended in patients who are overweight or obese.[19]

These suggestions are reasonable, of course. However, the vast majority of type 2 diabetics are on medication to manage their blood glucose levels. In fact, a survey conducted by the Centers for Disease Control from 1997 through 2011 reported that, in 2011, 17.7 million diabetics were on some kind of medication to manage their diabetes in the United States. Conversely, only 3.1 million diabetics reported managing their condition independent of drugs. Over five times as many diabetics were taking medication to manage their diabetes.

In 1997, the number of people taking any kind of medication to manage their diabetes was 8.4 million, while the number of people managing their diabetes independently was a mere 1.8 million. The number of people taking diabetes medication increased by 9.3 million people in 14 years, while the number of people taking care of their diabetes without drug assistance only increased by 1.3 million.[24]

Despite the claims that nutrition and weight management are the first lines of treatment for type 2 diabetes, the numbers show that an overwhelming majority of people rely on medication to manage their blood sugar. This is worrisome for a few key reasons:

- Medications do not slow the progression of diabetes.
- Medications do not "cure" diabetes, they just keep your blood sugar artificially low.
- Many diabetes medications come with long-term risks and consequences, such as an increased risk of heart attack.
- Sulfonylureas reduce your body's ability to produce insulin, making you more drug-dependent.
- People are taking drugs to counter the effects of poor diets, rather than change their eating habits.

Diabetes Medications

Metformin

There are dozens of options for a diabetic patient who may be prescribed medication. Metformin is one of the most common prescriptions for diabetes, and is often the first choice. It works by increasing tissue sensitivity to insulin. It also reduces the amount of glucose manufactured by the liver. Some side affects of metformin include diarrhea and nausea. The metformin may also fail to lower blood glucose effectively on its own.

If a patient's nutrition and exercise efforts also fail to be productive, the patient will likely be prescribed a secondary medication.[19]

Though it used to be rare, insulin has become a more popular choice for patients as a secondary medication. Due to its ability to give patients quick and easily accommodating blood glucose control, insulin began to be prescribed more often in conjunction with metformin over the last several years. However, research conducted by Dr. Christianne L. Roumie from the Veterans Health Administration-Tennessee Valley Healthcare System Geriatric Research Education Clinical Center, and Vanderbilt University, along with her colleagues, has suggested that the combination of metformin and insulin could be a quite lethal one. Study findings suggested that the use of metformin and insulin together increased the risks of cardiovascular events and possible mortality.25

Types of treatments conventional medicine suggests:

- Metformin
- Sulfonylureas
- Meglitinides
- Thiazolidinediones
- Insulin
- Bariatric surgery

The authors wrote, "Our finding of a modestly increased risk of a composite of cardiovascular events and death in metformin users who add insulin compared with sulfonylurea is consistent with the available clinical trial and observational data. None of these studies found an advantage of insulin compared with oral agents for cardiovascular risk, and several reported increased cardiovascular risk or weight gain and hypoglycemic episodes, which could result in poorer outcomes." The authors also call for further studies to continue to investigate the risks that may be associated with the use of insulin and metformin combined.[25]

Sulfonylureas

Sulfonylureas work by increasing the production of insulin by the pancreas. Some side affects include low blood sugar (hypoglycemia) and weight gain.[19] Gaining weight is the exact opposite of what a diabetic patient wants to do, as being overweight or obese is linked to the onset of the disease.

Sulfonylureas have been in use since the 1950s, and there are many different types. They all impose the same action, the stimulation of beta cells to release insulin, but the mechanism by which they generate this result result may differ, also lending to a variety of other potential side affects that may afflict the patient. [26]

Meglitinides

Meglitinides are another type of medication for diabetes that act through encouraging insulin production in the pancreas. However, meglitinides are faster acting than sulfonylureas. Their effects are also much more short lived in the body and run their course quickly. Meglitinides generally must be taken three times a day, before each meal. They also boast low blood sugar levels and potential weight gain as side effects. [19]

Thiazolidinesdiones

Thiazolidinediones act very similar to drugs like metformin by increasing tissue sensitivity to insulin. It is through this increased sensitivity that the cells are able to regain their ability to respond to insulin. However, thiazolidinediones are associated with weight gain and other, more critical risks. For example, thiazolidinediones have been shown increase the risk of heart failure or fracturing a bone. For this reason, they are not typically a first choice. [19]

Insulin

There are many other drugs on the marketplace for the treatment of type 2 diabetes. Insulin, for example, was once a last-resort measure for treatment of type 2 diabetes. Its use has grown in popularity, and it is often prescribed sooner due to its purported benefits. [19] Insulin can be prescribed to patients for basal or prandial (meal-time) use. It is common for patients to first be prescribed a long-acting basal injection of insulin before being prescribed faster-acting insulin for postprandial glucose control.

It is common for patients to prefer to have their basal injection increased as opposed to having prandial injections added to their daily prescription due to the convenience of doing so. However, it can be more detrimental to health, as it causes patients to never truly be in a fasting state. As such, their blood glucose never truly lowers appropriately after meals. In these cases, the basal insulin injection is essentially being used for postprandial management of blood sugar and it does not work in the same way as a basal injection in conjunction with prandial injections.[27] As previously noted, when insulin and metformin are used together, the patient's risk for a negative outcome, such as death, increases.[25]

When Drugs Aren't Enough

If medication isn't enough, MayoClinic.org also lists bariatric surgery as a potential treatment for type 2 diabetes. Major surgery with potential risk of fatality is a recommended treatment modality for patients with a BMI of 35 or greater.[19] That's a rather extreme course of action for a condition that can be treated with food and exercise.

The site states that in 55 to 95% of surgery recipients, blood glucose levels return to normal post-operation. The site also goes on to say that, in procedures where part of the small intestine is bypassed, the surgery's efficacy is more pronounced. Nowhere do they mention the fact that weight loss and new dietary requirements play a role in the alleviation from the symptoms of the disease.[19] Instead, they make it seem as though the surgery itself, and not the dietary changes and resulting weight loss that frequently accompany the surgery, are the reason for the positive outcomes.

It is also important to note that part of the recommended bariatric diet is the elimination of soda and other carbonated beverages, sweetened beverages and other sugar-laden items as well as refined grains and fatty foods. The suggested daily caloric intake for a person following the bariatric diet is 900 to 1,000 calories per day. The carbonation is eliminated so as not to harm the newly made stomach pouch or cause discomfort. Sugary or fatty foods are eliminated so as to keep caloric intake low, and to prevent dumping syndrome.

Dumping syndrome occurs when the stomach dumps food that has not been fully broken down into the small intestine. Symptoms of dumping syndrome include increased heart rate, diarrhea and vomiting. Portion control is also extremely important to limit the above symptoms, and to prevent stretching or tearing the stomach pouch.[28] Being overweight or obese, and keeping a diet laden with sugary foods and beverages, is positively associated with the onset of type 2 diabetes.[11] A diet high in saturated fats is also associated with the development of the disease.[6]

The bariatric diet conveniently forces a person to eliminate these causative factors from their diet, and promotes extreme weight loss by reducing a patient's capacity to eat larger portions of food, in addition to the reduction of calorie-dense sweets and fats along with recommending a very low daily calorie intake.[28] Reducing the intake of sweets and fats along with reducing total intake of calories each day is generally how people try to lose weight even without having major surgery, often in conjunction with exercise.

Why Conventional Treatment doesn't Work

Conventional treatment has several faults. First and foremost, patient compliance and adherence to a daily treatment schedule and meal plan can be difficult to achieve. In fact, a study conducted by Dr. David F. Blackburn, from the College of Pharmacy and Nutrition at the University of Saskatchewan, and his cohorts found that, on average, about 50% of newly diagnosed and prescribed diabetic patients will fail to take upwards of 80% of their medication in the first year. [29]

Another study, conducted by Anders Rosengren, MD, PhD, from the Department of Clinical Studies at Lund University in Sweden, along with his colleagues, found that sulfonylurea treatment will eventually fail and results in all patients needing to take injectable insulin therapy as well in order to manage blood sugar levels. This condition is referred to as "secondary failure," and develops within just a few years of treatment with the medication.

The explanation behind this is that sulfonylureas stimulate the pancreatic beta cells to produce more insulin. Eventually, these beta cells become exhausted and are no longer able to produce enough insulin, even with more of the stimulation drugs. The end result is that the patient becomes dependent on injectable insulin for treatment of their diabetes.

One popular hypothesis is that the sulfonylurea-induced excitation of the beta cells can create an excitotoxic reaction, and eventually leads to decreased beta cell mass in the pancreas. The researchers also noted that clinical experience did not suggest that the cessation of the sulfonylurea medication would result in the return of normal beta cell function in patients that had developed secondary failure.[30]

The drugs prescribed to treat diabetes often increase body weight and other health risks that encourage the development of type 2 diabetes.[19] Continuing to absorb glucose when it isn't warranted can eventually kill the cell.[31]

The logic behind these medications is generally that, if the blood sugar is lower, the patient must be getting healthier, even if their weight is climbing upwards and they were overweight to begin with. What causes the weight gain? The medication is essentially forcing the body to absorb sugar from the blood – and store it as fat. Cell refusal to uptake glucose is not necessarily a malfunction. It can also be a defense mechanism. You can see where a medication forcing the cells to accept glucose that isn't needed could cause potential problems.

It is also imperative to realize that insulin resistance does not act alone. Leptin is a hormone that lets your brain know when you don't need to continue eating. When your body is unable to store excess glucose, insulin triggers the production of triglycerides. These triglycerides can block the reception of leptin in the brain, causing you to keep eating even though you don't actually need to. This in turn perpetuates high blood sugar levels and weight gain.

As the process repeats day in and day out, insulin resistance develops and turns into type 2 diabetes, along with other conditions such as high triglycerides, high blood pressure and high cholesterol. The pattern of disease is set, and is continued by the prescribed medications that make a patient dependent on an ever-increasing dosage to keep their bodies in a barely functioning state.[31]

Managing diabetes: Medicine VS. Diet

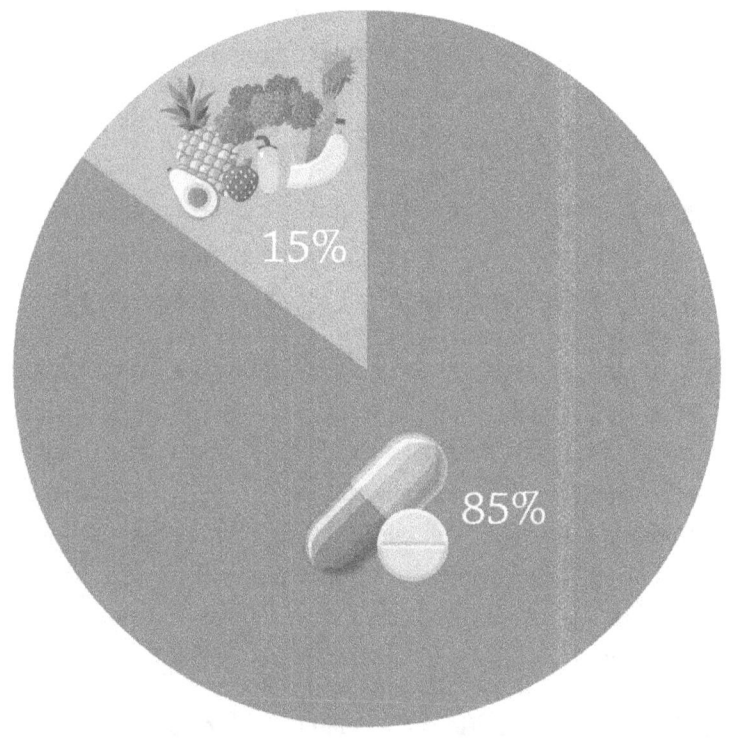

15%

85%

Out of 20.8 million people with diabetes, 17.7 million manage diabetes with medicine, while

only 3.1 million people manage diabetes with a healthy diet

Dietary changes are the most common suggestion made by doctors, dietitians and holistic health professionals. The difference is what's being suggested. A typical diabetic diet prescribed in medical nutrition therapy (MNT) consists of three meals and one to three snacks a day, depending on the patient's calorie and lifestyle needs. In a conventional diabetic meal plan, the patient would divide their allotted carbohydrates relatively evenly across the day.

For example, if a patient were allowed 120 grams of carbohydrates, that patient may choose to have 30 grams for their three main meals, and two snacks containing 15 grams each. Carbohydrate counting and dispersion throughout the day is supposed to help diabetics maintain their blood sugar levels on an even keel throughout the day. It is also supposed to help prevent or delay the many common but dreadful side affects of diabetes that has not been managed, such as toe, foot or leg amputation or kidney damage.

The general suggestion by doctors and dietitians is that carbohydrates should make up 45 to 65% of your daily caloric intake. They suggest whole grains, fruits and vegetables should be your first choice foods, but a carbohydrate-counting diet doesn't really differentiate between whole wheat bread and candy. It assumes all carbohydrate sources essentially have the same effect on the body, with some sources being more nutrient- or calorie-dense than others or higher in carbohydrates per serving.[32]

However, the glycemic index suggests the theory that all carbohydrates are created equal in terms of their effect on your blood sugar is incorrect. The glycemic index rates foods on a scale of 0–100, based on the extent to which they raise blood sugar levels after consumption. Foods with high glycemic indexes are associated with rapid digestion and fast absorption, which lead to noticeable fluctuations in blood glucose levels after consumption. Conversely, foods with low glycemic indexes are associated with slower digestion and absorption and a more gradual and steady rise and fall of blood sugar levels post-meal. Low glycemic index diets have been shown to improve blood glucose and lipid levels in patients with both type 1 and type 2 diabetes.[33]

As the University of Sydney states, "Foods with a high GI are those which are rapidly digested, absorbed and metabolised and result in marked fluctuations in blood sugar (glucose) levels. Low GI carbohydrates – the ones that produce smaller fluctuations in your blood glucose and insulin levels – is one of the secrets to long-term health, reducing your risk of type 2 diabetes and heart disease. It is also one of the keys to maintaining weight loss."[33]

In the case of a conventional carbohydrate-counting diabetic diet, it is still up to the patient to make better choices in regard to their food. A patient who follows the diet but is still eating white bread and donuts is not going to experience a high level of improvement, based on the evidence suggested by the glycemic index.

The conventional diet for diabetics proposed by MNT also fails in regard to overall blood glucose management. It is routine for even healthy people to be told that eating smaller, more frequent meals and snacks is better for them. This is perhaps something that has perpetuated the rise of type 2 diabetes across the nation. In normal, healthy individuals, insulin levels return to their basal status about three hours after a meal.

This is when your pancreas begins the production of glucagon, which is a hormone that stimulates the liver to release its glycogen stores. This process allows your body to naturally sustain its blood sugar levels with stored energy. Your liver is able to burn off its fat stores and make room for new storage the next time you eat, while also clearing excess triglycerides from your bloodstream. When this system is interfered with, such as with constant snacking, the release of glucagon to stimulate the liver is halted. Your liver doesn't release its energy stores, and insulin will be unable to deliver more glucose to the liver.

So where does the glucose go, if it can't be accepted by the liver? Well, first it circulates through your bloodstream, raising your blood sugar levels while insulin triggers your cells to accept more glucose stores. Eventually, this all leads to the body turning the excess glucose into fat. As your body weight rises, so do your chances of developing further insulin resistance. You may also develop a fatty liver over time, which carries with it a whole host of its own issues.[31] Many type 2 diabetics are prescribed a medication regimen to coincide with their conventional nutrition therapy to maximize the amount of glucose that will be absorbed after meals so the patients can obtain lower blood sugar levels.[32]

Between the effects of medication and a meal plan that prevents natural dips in blood glucose to stimulate the release of glycogen from the liver, it makes perfect sense as to why diabetes patients have such a hard time managing their condition with conventional therapy. There is nowhere for the glucose being consumed to be stored, other than as fat – resulting in weight gain, further insulin resistance and the continuation of disease. [32]

Conventional pharmacological solutions and medical nutrition therapy for diabetics fail to truly treat the cause of the disease. Instead, they focus on managing the symptoms. High blood sugar levels are the symptom of something sinister going on inside your body, also known as insulin resistance and leptin resistance. The byproducts of conventional therapies do not actually correct these issues. Most prescription medications for type 2 diabetes carry with them the probability of weight gain along with the chance of developing other conditions. MNT for type 2 diabetics often has negative implications for the patient as well. Most importantly, the frequent meals prescribed often result in the body never depleting its glycogen stores throughout the day, resulting in an inability to use new glucose that's been introduced to the bloodstream.[31]

Extreme suggestions, such as bariatric surgery, are often recommended as well, especially for obese patients. It is very frightening to live in a world where people think it is better to go under the knife to lose weight and have a doctor "fix" them, than to take responsibility for their own life.[19] The American people are overly reliant on prescriptions and doctors to make their ailments more tolerable, and it is a system that is self-perpetuating.[31]

People afflicted by type 2 diabetes cannot get better when doctors are prescribing medications that eventually make them even more dependent.[30] Mainstream medicine wants people to believe that there is no cure for type 2 diabetes, but that is simply not true. There is hope for managing and even reversing the condition, if you are willing to put in the work.

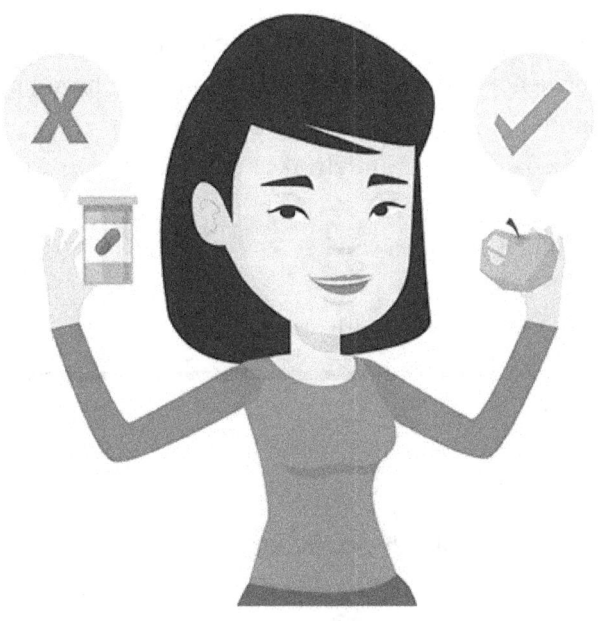

Chapter 3 – Type 2 Diabetes is Preventable and Treatable

There are many options for overcoming diabetes without medication. In fact, type 2 diabetes is actually one of the most preventable and readily treatable diseases out there, despite what conventional medicine would like you to believe. The Mayo Clinic website states right in their definition of type 2 diabetes that there is no cure, but it may be managed with diet and medication "if necessary."[2]

Diabetes can be prevented through a number of lifestyle and dietary modifications:

- Exercise more often
- Eat a nutritious diet that focuses on whole foods
- Avoid deficiency in key nutrients like vitamin D, chromium and magnesium
- Avoid sugar-laden foods and drinks (and high-fructose corn syrup)
- Quit smoking if you are a smoker
- Don't drink to excess
- Achieve and maintain a healthy body weight

Technically speaking, while the condition can be reversed, it cannot be cured. You can remove your risk for the development of diabetes complications and have consistently normal blood glucose levels, lipid profiles and blood pressure. But, if you start eating donuts and soda daily, you are likely going to be a type 2 diabetic again, because you have the pathology to develop the condition on a cellular level. That's why the condition can be reversed, but not cured at this time.[34]

Let's not forget how many millions more are on medication than those who are not. Fourteen million more Americans take drugs in an attempt to remedy this very treatable condition than those who have managed it independently.[24] That is no small margin of difference. It is a frighteningly great disparity. Still, most patients on diabetic medication will eventually find that their medication will fail them. Metformin often cannot treat diabetes on its own and needs to be used in conjunction with another medication.[19] Sulfonylureas have been proven to fail over time and require the patient to take insulin injections.[30]

The truth is that there are many natural, holistic options for the person who wants to truly reverse their type 2 diabetes diagnosis and repair their body. Not many people want to believe that because conventional medicine has brainwashed society into believing that these conditions caused by what we eat and how we live are irreversible and require medication to be "controlled."

Furthermore, most of these medications serve only to lower blood sugar. They do nothing to impede or cease the progression of the disease and its associated complications. In some instances, the prescribed drugs can actually accelerate the development of diabetes complications.[35] As an example, it is well documented that diabetes medications like metformin can cause patients to gain weight.[19]

This medication is also shown to increase the risk of cardiovascular events (such as heart attacks) and death in patients who receive it in conjunction with insulin injections. The metformin and insulin combination is not an unusual one, either. The addition of insulin became popular due to its ability to make controlling one's blood sugar more a thing of whimsy that required less structure and inconvenience.[25]

There is a difference between having a condition be "controlled," having it "reversed" and being "cured." Medications artificially control the patient's blood glucose levels. Even though the condition is being managed, the long-term effects of diabetes, such as blindness and kidney damage, do not cease to progress and develop.

When the condition is controlled by artificial means, its progression and development in the body still continues, but the symptom of high blood sugar levels is diminished, at least for a time.[34] Studies indicate that, over time, popular diabetes drugs cease to function.[30]

In reversal though, the condition has been more than just controlled or stopped through dietary intervention or medication. It's more than just having blood sugar levels consistently be within a normal range, along with other key markers such as blood pressure and cholesterol levels. It's your body being repaired at a cellular level, where the progression of the disease and its complications have been halted and damage that had been created has been undone. This repair and reversal cannot be completed with artificial means such as medication and requires a healthy diet filled with nutrients to conduct cellular repair.

Holistic medicine is whole body medicine. Some holistic approaches to treating diabetes may include:

- Dietary modifications
- Lifestyle changes
- Increase physical activity
- Juicing
- Supplementation

Homeopathic doctors also believe in a number of alternative therapies:

- Ayurvedic medicine
- Aromatherapy
- Chinese medicine
- Acupuncture
- Biofeedback

However, your experience with these treatments may vary. DiabetesScience.news is also a great resource for learning more about alternative therapies for diabetes, and more.

Reversal does require dietary and lifestyle maintenance to be sustained. Going back to bad habits will result in another onset of type 2 diabetes. To be "cured" of type 2 diabetes would indicate that a patient no longer carries the pathology for the disease at a cellular level. In other words, a patient could go back to drinking soda and not experience diabetic side effects. Though no cure has been announced yet, that does not mean it is not out there.[34]

Changing your diet and lifestyle are the most significant changes you can make in order to reverse type 2 diabetes. Diet and exercise are everything when it comes to this condition. What you eat and how you live can change your life for the better. The U.S. government's Third National Health and Nutrition Examination Survey (NHANES III) found that 69% of diabetics either did not engage in physical activity regularly or did not exercise at all; 62% ate fewer than five servings of fruits and vegetables a day; and 82% were overweight or obese.[35] Keeping a poor diet, having a low physical activity level and being overweight or obese are three primary environmental factors in the onset of type 2 diabetes.[1]

It is not really that surprising that so many people with the condition appear to be making less than concentrated efforts towards healing their bodies. After all, the doctor always says that's what medication is for. Why do patients need to exercise or eat better if they can take drugs instead?

Scientific Evidence in the Reversal of Type 2 Diabetes

A study conducted by the Diabetes Prevention Program found that 150 minutes of physical activity such as brisk walking, or activities of similar intensity, reduced the risk of developing type 2 diabetes by 58%. This same study also looked at early exposure to drug therapy with metformin as a potential preventative care method. Early use of metformin only provided a 31% reduction in risk for developing type 2 diabetes. Walking alone was nearly twice as efficacious at reducing the risks for the onset of type 2 diabetes as a common prescription drug.[35] It has also been previously documented that metformin often fails to induce enough tissue sensitivity on its own and may frequently require a secondary medication to be prescribed over time.[19] Exercise is a much better option because it won't require you to take an ever-increasing amount of prescription medications.

Though physical activity is of great importance in the treatment and prevention of type 2 diabetes, exercise by itself is not enough. A new study published by the *Journal of Epidemiology* suggests that being obese cannot be compensated for with physical fitness. The study began analyzing over 1 million Swedish men who were about 18 years of age between 1966 and 1996. They were followed until their death or the study's end in 2012. The researchers' findings were that obese men in the highest fifth of physical fitness were still at a higher risk of mortality than normal-weight men regardless of their physical fitness, or unfitness as the case may be.[36] It is not enough to just add exercise to your daily regime if you seek to reduce your risk of death and disease. A healthy diet and a healthy weight are imperative in the quest to change your life. Being overweight or obese is still one of the primary risk factors in the onset of type 2 diabetes.[1]

The fact is that changing one aspect of your life without reducing your weight or changing your diet is simply not enough. This study also found that the more obese a person was, the higher their risk of mortality and disease was, regardless of how physically fit the person may have been.[36] Being healthy is cyclical. Participating in one singular aspect of a healthy life does not inherently mean you are healthy.

The goals of natural medicine in the treatment of type 2 diabetes are to bring about consistently normal blood glucose levels and to achieve ideal metabolic status and regular function of insulin and other hormones. Natural treatment also seeks to reduce the risks associated with type 2 diabetes and improve cholesterol, blood pressure and other health markers.

Through nutrition, holistic medicine is able to provide optimal micronutrient consumption for healing, reduce postprandial blood sugar elevations, improve insulin function and sensitivity, and prevent oxidative stress.[35] Dietary modifications can also help reduce weight. Obesity is associated with the kind of damaging inflammation that may predicate insulin resistance and type 2 diabetes.[6] The inclusion of high-fiber, low-sugar foods that are nutrient-dense but low in calories can help reduce weight and the inflammation associated with obesity. Following a healthier diet and losing weight can also reduce your blood sugar levels.[37]

A 2010 study published in the *Archives of Internal Medicine* concluded that making significant lifestyle and dietary changes yielded much more promising results for patients than did medication alone. In fact, the lifestyle changes not only improved the patients' diabetes but also reduced their risks for cardiovascular disease. The researchers agreed that diet and exercise were indeed a better option for patients based on their results. Two different treatment protocols were analyzed in the study of over 5,000 obese patients with type 2 diabetes, over a four-year period. The first group of patients was treated with an "intensive lifestyle intervention" program that included new dietary regimens and physical fitness programs. The second group received medication and met three times a year for an education and support group.[38]

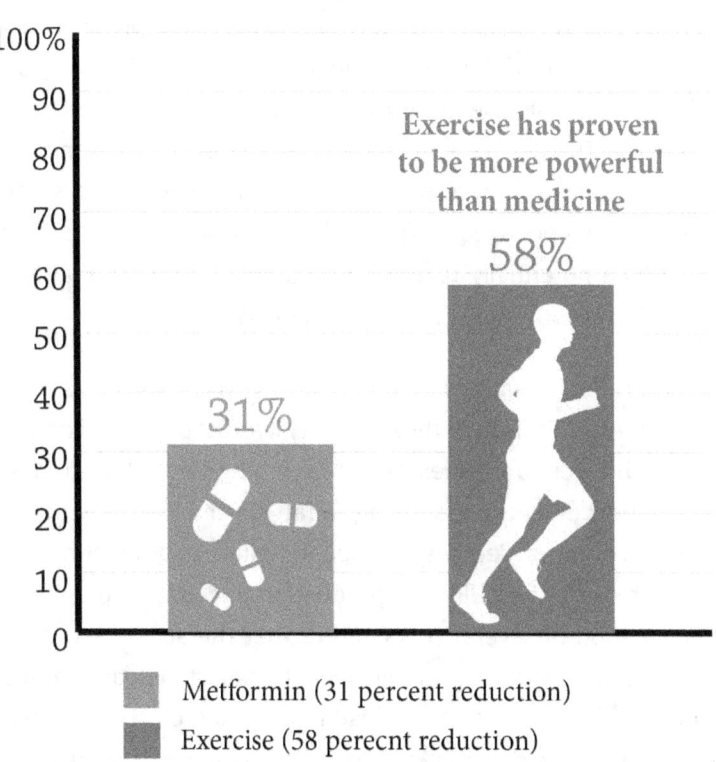

Reducing diabetes risk

Exercise has proven to be more powerful than medicine

58%

31%

Metformin (31 percent reduction)
Exercise (58 perecnt reduction)

At the end of the four-year period, the lifestyle intervention group had averaged a loss of more than 6% of their total starting body weight, while the medication group had averaged less than 1%. The lifestyle intervention group also experienced better A1C levels, which is a long-term measure of blood glucose, lower blood pressure and better cholesterol profiles. Medication does precious little for patients suffering from type 2 diabetes, and this study suggests that lifestyle changes should be the primary focus of those who wish to reverse their condition and improve their overall health. The journey to a healthy body begins with achieving a healthy weight, consuming healthy foods and making time for physical activity.[38]

A 2013 study authored by Dr. Roy Taylor from the Institute of Cellular Medicine at Newcastle University in the United Kingdom concluded that fasting plasma glucose levels can normalize within seven days of the introduction of a substantially low-calorie diet. Dr. Taylor posits that this rapid change is related to the substantial decrease in liver fat stores, which is then followed by the return of hepatic insulin sensitivity. In other words, a very low-calorie diet prompts the liver to use up its glycogen stores, which are made of glucose. The decrease in glycogen stores encourages insulin sensitivity in the liver tissue to return to normal, as it has room to accept new glucose from the blood stream. The author suggests that type 2 diabetes can be seen as a potentially reversible metabolic condition that has been hastened by chronic, excess fat within the bodily organs.[39]

Dr. Taylor also refers to what is called the "twin cycle hypothesis of etiology of type 2 diabetes." In this hypothesis, a fatty liver leads to a secondary fatty pancreas, which leads to a series of self-repeating cycles that brings about the onset of type 2 diabetes. Essentially, a fatty liver will experience a rise in insulin resistance and a decrease of hepatic glucose production. This will lead to an increase in basal insulin production and fasting plasma glucose levels over a period of several years and further the accumulation of fat in the liver. Over time, the fatty liver will begin to export increased amounts of very low-density lipid triacylglycerol, leading to an increase of fat deposits in all tissues, including the pancreatic islets, where beta cells produce insulin.

It is expected that an excess of fatty acids in the pancreatic tissue would impair the beta cells' ability to produce insulin efficiently. The findings of this study support the concept of the twin cycle theory in that they suggest there is a maximum tolerance to fatty acid levels in the liver and pancreas, and exceeding this tolerance may trigger the onset of type 2 diabetes. The supporting evidence is that, when these fat levels dropped, the subjects' insulin sensitivity returned to normal.[39]

There is likely a genetic factor that affects different individuals' level of tolerance to fatty acids in their organs. But this does not change the fact that, if a person has type 2 diabetes, it is likely that they have too much fat in their liver and pancreas.[39]

Dr. Taylor also went on to write, "Type 2 diabetes has long been regarded as inevitably progressive, requiring increasing numbers of oral hypoglycemic agents and eventually insulin, but it is now certain that the disease process can be halted with restoration of normal carbohydrate and fat metabolism."[39]

Type 2 diabetes often progresses in spite of medication, leading upwards of 50% of patients requiring insulin therapy within 10 years. This level of deterioration has caused many people to believe that, while it is treatable, it is not curable. Dr. Taylor's research supports the belief that, with dietary changes and weight loss, type 2 diabetes can in fact be reversed.[39]

It may seem easier to just take a medication to "control" your condition, but the evidence is very clear – taking pills doesn't make you better; it just prolongs the inevitable. The only path to health is one that requires effort and personal responsibility. There is no immediate remedy to type 2 diabetes. It takes time to truly heal your body from the damage incurred by this condition, and what caused it. There is no vitamin you can take or a pill you can swallow that will "make it all better" overnight.

What you need to do to reverse type 2 diabetes is create a healthier internal and external environment for yourself.[31] As previously noted, it has been proven in numerous studies such as Dr. Taylor's and the one performed by the Diabetes Prevention Program that lifestyle changes including diet and exercise promote the reversal of type 2 diabetes. Other studies have proven that medication does very little to improve the condition for patients long-term.[30]

How Holistic Nutrition Can Help

Perhaps one of the most important conclusions that can be drawn from all of this is that high blood sugar is merely a symptom of the disease – and not the disease itself. Conventional medicine is so caught up with micromanaging this one symptom that the rest of the disease is overlooked. Some may say this where conventionalists fail to see the forest for the trees. Too narrow a focus often yields poor results, and this is especially true in medicine. Conventional medicine focuses on the symptom of insulin resistance – high blood sugar – and seeks to manage this symptom. Conventional medicine fails to look at what is causing this insulin resistance. Though conventional medicine may put diabetes under a microscope – it is exactly this that prevents them from seeing the whole picture.

There are many supplements that may help with diabetes:

- Astaxanthin
- Probiotics
- Turmeric
- Fish oil
- Chia seeds
- Whey protein
- Magnesium
- Selenium

You can learn more about the benefits of these items and more in Chapter 6.

Holistic medicine focuses on the health of the entire body, and remembers that the body is a complete system that functions best in harmony. If one organ fails, the rest will eventually fail also. One of the core philosophies of holistic medicine is that it is important to heal the cause of the disease, and not just mediate the symptoms.[40] Mainstream diabetes treatment does the exact opposite of that. The sole purpose of diabetes medication is not to remedy the disease, but to manage the symptom of high blood sugar.[19]

This does very little for the patient's long-term outcome.

There are dozens of options for the person who wants to truly reverse their type 2 diabetes that don't involve going to the doctor to get a prescription medication and insulin injections. To begin, exercise is an obvious must. With physical activity, the body is able to use its glycogen stores found in muscle tissue, increasing their insulin sensitivity and preparing them to accept glucose from the blood stream. Exercise also burns energy and lowers your risk of becoming overweight, along with reducing your risk for many other diseases.[9]

Diet is another primary factor in the reversal of type 2 diabetes. There are many opinions on the correct diet a type 2 diabetic should be following. The diet recommended by the conventional medical establishment contains mostly whole grains, fruits, vegetables, lean proteins and low-fat dairy products. Many alternative nutrition therapists suggest that eliminating grains may be beneficial to patients, because grains elicit a higher glycemic response than other carbohydrate sources. Minimally processed foods, like sweet potatoes, may be emphasized over convenience items like bread. Some also feel that grains contain components that can be irritating and contribute to inflammation, such as gluten.[41]

Conventionalists suggest that diabetics eat a minimal amount of fat per day, along with obtaining less than 7% of their dietary fat from saturated fats; it is also suggested that they keep their cholesterol at or below 200mg per day. However, holistic nutritionists feel that low-fat is going in the entirely wrong direction. Fat is a necessary part of every meal to mediate the glycemic response and slow the digestion and absorption of food, to promote slow and steady blood glucose levels. Good, wholesome fats from whole dairy products, egg yolks, fatty fish, nuts, avocados and the like are not considered to be bad for you. Trans fats and added fats found in processed foods are what you should avoid, according to holistic nutritionists.[41]

Fiber and protein are also considered important parts of the diet in both nutrition ideologies. However, in holistic nutrition, certain protein sources are heartily recommended, such as wild-caught fatty fish. In conventional therapy, a patient is generally recommended to get 25 to 30 grams of fiber per day through whole grains, cereals, fruits and vegetables. In holistic nutrition, it is common to suggest patients eat eight to ten servings of fruit and vegetables per day so they get the added benefits of all the phytonutrients and micronutrients found in produce.

In general, the holistic approach to nutrition advocates whole, natural foods as opposed to more processed foods in conjunction with a diet that is generally lower in carbohydrates, and higher in fat, protein, fiber and micronutrients, than a conventionally prescribed diet.[41]

A number of supplements in the form of vitamins, minerals and herbs have also been discovered to help alleviate the symptoms of type 2 diabetes, and help bring about its reversal.

It is not individually by which these things are able to help reverse diabetes, but rather, collectively. It is the combination of effort on all fronts by which a person can regain their freedom from disease and reverse their diagnosis of type 2 diabetes.

Chapter 4 – Foods To Eat Or Avoid For Reversing Type 2 Diabetes

To begin our discussion of diet, it is important to go over the different types of nutrients and their roles in their body. From there, we can better understand how these nutrients impact diabetics, and what roles they can play in recovery from the condition.

There are three macronutrients – carbohydrates, protein and fat – which provide energy, or calories, and are required for growth, metabolism and most other bodily functions. Macronutrients are named as such because they are required in large quantities.

The basic function of carbohydrates is to provide energy for the body. Protein is primarily used for growth and repair, but can also be used for energy when carbohydrate sources are not available. Fat is necessary for normal growth and development, the maintenance of cell membranes and the absorption of several key vitamins and minerals. Micronutrients are nutrients that are required in smaller amounts, like vitamins and minerals. Together, macronutrients, micronutrients and water provide the essentials needed to sustain life.[42]

Phytonutrients are a type of phytochemical ("plant chemical") found in plants that influence plant health. There are hundreds of phytonutrients, many unique to specific colors of fruits and vegetables. Many phytonutrients have also been found to provide health benefits to humans, such as scavenging free radicals or fighting bacterial infections.[43]

Nutrition is imperative to leading a healthy life. There is no better way to prevent disease and heal your body than through food. The basics of the diet suggested for type 2 diabetic individuals is that they should consume a diet rich in fruits and vegetables, fiber, healthy fats and protein. The diet should also be low in or eliminate refined grains such as white bread, sugar-sweetened beverages, trans fats and sweets.[44]

Foods to Avoid at All Costs

There are many foods that should be avoided, but especially in the case of a type 2 diabetic. Processed and added sugars, like high-fructose corn syrup, are not good for anyone, but if you are a type 2 diabetic seeking to reverse your condition, it is of utmost importance to divorce yourself from sugar-sweetened treats and processed foods. Most processed foods contain some form of added sugar for flavor enhancement, even if they don't taste sweet. All of these added sugars cause extreme peaks and falls in blood glucose levels.

This is not good for anyone, but is especially bad for people who already have type 2 diabetes, as it just exacerbates the condition. Sugar-sweetened beverages have the same negative impact on blood sugar levels and should also be avoided.[44]

Foods to avoid (and enjoy) to fight diabetes:
- Processed foods of any kind
- Refined grains
- Added sugars, including high fructose corn syrup
- Added fats, including trans fats
- Artificial sweeteners
- "Reduced fat" foods
- Sugar-sweetened beverages

Foods to Enjoy:
- Fruits and vegetables
- Whole grains
- Beans and legumes
- Nuts and seeds
- Wild-caught fatty fish
- Pasture-raised meat and poultry

The Glycemic Index

These items can also be classified as "high-glycemic-index foods" in addition to being foods laced with added sugars. High-glycemic-index foods may also include items made from white flour or white rice. Even though these items may not have added sugars, they are low in fiber, fat and protein but high in carbohydrates. As such, the carbohydrates are quickly and readily digested, broken down into glucose and absorbed into the blood stream, which creates a spike in blood sugar levels. Foods that carry a high-glycemic-index should generally be avoided, especially if they are low in nutrient value – which is the case for white flour products.[33]

High-glycemic-index foods are not always high in glycemic load though. The difference between glycemic index and glycemic load is that the index refers to a food's effect on blood sugar when a certain number of carbohydrates have been obtained from that food. It is the equivalent of comparing 25 grams of carbohydrate from a slice of bread to 25 grams of carbohydrate in 5 cups of broccoli. How often do you eat 5 cups of broccoli at once though? That is the question glycemic load serves to answer by ranking foods not by their effect on blood sugar levels in a given carbohydrate quantity, but rather based on the amount of carbohydrates in a normal serving of food. So a food that is high on the glycemic index but low in glycemic load – like a banana – is not inherently bad for you, especially because bananas are nutrient-dense and a good source of fiber. Using glycemic load and glycemic index for food choices still requires common sense. Bacon does not have a notable glycemic value, but it is not something you should eat at every meal.[45]

Trans Fats

Trans fat is another ingredient to be wary of. Excess trans fat intake has been shown to increase the incidence of type 2 diabetes.[44] Trans fats have also been found to increase the levels of LDL cholesterol in your blood stream. There are two types of trans fat. The first is a naturally occurring trans fat that can be found in the gut of some grazing animals, like cows. The second type of trans fat is man-made. Trans fats are man-made fats synthesized from plant fats. Plant fats, such as olive oil, tend to be liquid at room temperature. Through chemical alteration to the structure of the fatty acid chains, trans fats were born, and suddenly we had plant fats that were solid at room temperate – like margarine.[46] For a time, these were believed to be better than traditional solid fats like butter.[44]

It is also important to remember that, per the FDA, trans fats need only be reported on a nutrition label if the product carries more than half a gram of trans fat per serving. So, that pastry you bought at the gas station may be considered four servings, and each serving may have up to a half a gram of trans fats. That's two grams of trans fat hidden in just one product! If you see partially hydrogenated oils on a food label, it contains trans fats and you probably shouldn't eat it.[46]

Trans fats can hide in any number of foods, so it is important to check ingredient labels for key words like "partially hydrogenated oils." Some common places trans fat can hide are:

- Frozen foods
- Prepackaged foods
- Any kind of processed food item
- Coffee creamer
- Pastries and other bakery goods

It is also important to remember that, per the FDA, trans fats need only be reported on a nutrition label if the product carries more than half a gram of trans fat per serving. So, that pastry you bought at the gas station may be considered four servings, and each serving may have up to a half a gram of trans fats. That's two grams of trans fat hidden in just one product! If you see partially hydrogenated oils on a food label, it contains trans fats and you probably shouldn't eat it.[46]

Reduced-Fat Foods

It has long been suggested that type 2 diabetics should follow a low-fat diet. However, a study headed by Dr. Maiorino Esposito of the Second University of Naples Department of Geriatrics and Metabolic Diseases compared long-term outcomes of patients that followed the typically prescribed low-fat diet, patients that followed a Mediterranean diet that was higher in healthy fats and patients prescribed a low-carbohydrate diet. The diets were assigned randomly to the test subjects. The test subjects met with dietitians and nutritionists once a month the first year, and once every other month in the following years. At the end of the four-year study period, some interesting findings were to be had.

The test group that followed the conventional low-fat diabetic diet ended up with 70% of its participants requiring daily prescription drugs to manage their blood sugar levels. Less than half of the Mediterranean group required any type of medication related to their type 2 diabetes at all. The Mediterranean group also had a significant decrease in their risk factors for cardiovascular disease, and they lost more weight than their low-fat counterparts, despite not having any increase in physical activity levels. These findings suggest that dietary fat, specifically monounsaturated fats, can have a very positive role in the management and reversal of type 2 diabetes.[47] This makes sense when you consider that a lot of reduced-fat items have added sugars, sugar substitutes and other additives like corn starch to make up for the loss of flavor and texture when fat is removed. [48]

Processed Foods, Sugars and Artificial Sweeteners

Processed foods are truly one of the biggest culprits in the rise of death and disease in today's world. This is especially true of type 2 diabetes, as it is greatly promoted by the excessive intake of added fats and sugars. The sodium nitrates and nitrites found in processed meats in particular have been found to be toxic to humans and can incite the growth of cancer cells. Nitrates and nitrites have also been linked to the onset of many diseases, including type 2 diabetes.

In fact, a study published in 2010 in the journal *Circulation* found that regular consumption of just two ounces a day of processed meat led to a 20% increased risk for developing diabetes. For this reason, processed meats such as hot dogs, deli meat and other preserved meats and items that contain nitrates or nitrites should be avoided.[49]

In addition to added sugars, trans fats and sodium nitrate and nitrite, what else should be avoided? Diet soda. Numerous studies have shown that diet sodas are no good, but did you know that they have actually been attributed to several components of metabolic syndrome and type 2 diabetes? In fact, a study published by the American Diabetes Association found that there was a 67% increased risk for developing type 2 diabetes among people who regularly consumed diet beverages as compared to those who did not consume diet soda at all. The study, which used data from the Multi-Ethnic Study of Atherosclerosis, also found that regularly drinking diet soda correlated with a waist circumference higher than 100 centimeters.[50]

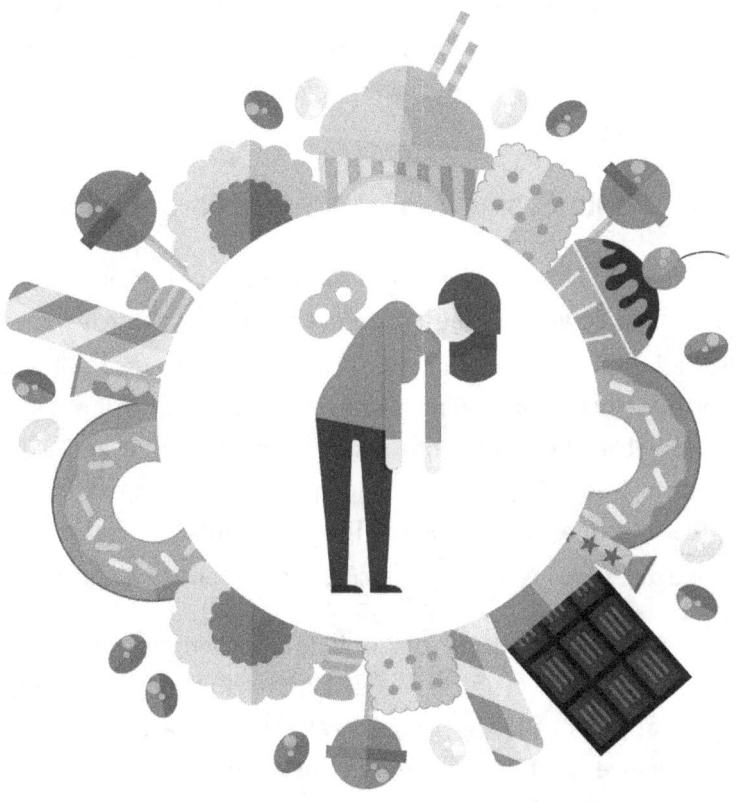

A recent study published in the journal *Nature* also detailed how artificial sweeteners such as aspartame and sucralose raise the risk for developing type 2 diabetes, and alter the bacteria and homeostasis of a healthy gut. The findings of their study suggest that glucose intolerance was induced through alterations in the gut bacteria, precipitated by the consumption of artificial sweeteners.[51]

So, what is a type 2 diabetic supposed to eat then?

Type 2 Diabetic Nutrition Basics

Fruits and vegetables should be the primary source of carbohydrates for a type 2 diabetic, along with whole grains. Fruits and vegetables are rich in key vitamins, minerals and phytonutrients. This makes them very nutrient-dense choices that also happen to be fairly low in calories (with a few exceptions). Whole grains are excellent grain choices compared to bleached and processed options.

Choosing Whole Grains and Low-Sugar Carbohydrates

Whole grains are higher in fiber and have a much better nutrient profile. Fiber helps slow down the digestion process, as most fiber is indigestible and poses a bit of a challenge to your body to break down.[43] Fiber can be soluble or insoluble. Soluble fiber dissolves in water, while insoluble fiber does not. Soluble fiber turns into a gel during digestion and slows the process down. Insoluble fiber can help speed up the expedition of food through the intestines. Both types of fiber are equally important in maintaining good digestive health and reducing and preventing disease.[52]

Researcher Anne Nilsson from the Unit for Applied Nutrition and Food Chemistry at Lund University in Sweden found that the consumption of whole grains as part of a low-glycemic breakfast encouraged better memory skills and cognitive function in addition to better blood sugar levels. In fact, the low-glycemic breakfast with whole grains was found to stabilize blood sugar levels for up to 10 hours. But was it just the whole grains, or was it the low-glycemic breakfast? Nilsson's results concluded that those who ate the low-glycemic index breakfast were found to have much better cognition than the test subjects who ate a high-glycemic-index breakfast. Nilsson also suggests that people with greater fluctuations in blood sugar levels run a greater risk for having a generally lower cognitive ability. In other words, eating poor quality food degrades not just your body but also your brain as well.[53] Whole grains or other low-glycemic-index carbohydrate sources such as fruits, vegetables, beans and legumes are all excellent choices for the type 2 diabetic.

Wild-Caught Fatty Fish

Fish, particularly wild-caught fatty fish like salmon, are an excellent protein choice for type 2 diabetics. Why? For one, the omega-3 fatty acids found in fatty fish help to lower triglycerides in the bloodstream.[54] If you recall from Chapter 2, when there is excess glucose in the bloodstream, insulin may trigger the production of triglycerides. These triglycerides can block the reception of leptin in the brain, and the cycle of overeating, insulin resistance and high blood glucose levels repeats itself.[31] The consumption of omega-3s can help reduce the number of these harmful triglycerides traveling in your blood stream, and expedite the healing process.[54] Fish such as wild-caught salmon also tend to be an excellent source of vitamin D. Poor control of blood glucose levels and the onset of type 2 diabetes may be predicated by vitamin D deficiency. The consumption of foods rich in this vital nutrient, like fatty fish, mushrooms and almonds, can help promote better blood glucose control.[10]

Protein for Blood Sugar Control

New research presented in 2015 at the annual meeting for the European Association for the Study of Diabetes suggested that a higher-protein diet may help promote better blood glucose control. Over a period of six weeks, 37 participants were fed either a diet high in animal protein or a diet high in plant protein. The animal protein group received both meat and cheese, while the plant protein group received strictly vegan meals. Both groups received the same number of calories per day. Both groups saw a decrease in blood sugar levels and fatty tissue in their livers. However, only the animal protein group saw an increase in their insulin sensitivity. Conversely, the plant protein group showed improved kidney function. This study has shown that plant protein may be easier on the kidneys for diabetics who may be at risk for or have already developed diabetic kidney disease.[55] Both lean meats that are pasture-raised and wholesome sources of plant protein like lentils should be included as part of a healthy diet for a type 2 diabetic. Some plant proteins, such as beans and legumes, also contain carbohydrates so that should be taken into account when planning a meal.

A Basic Summary of Nutrition for Type 2 Diabetes

The core of basic nutrition in regard to type 2 diabetes revolves around the elimination of processed foods, high-sugar and high-fat items, foods containing added sugars and trans fats and white flour or other processed and refined grain products from the diet. It is imperative to replace these non-nutritive items with nutrient-dense foods such as fruits, vegetables, nuts, seeds and whole grains. Lean meats and fish may also be included in the diet as well. Consuming more fiber and nutrients and less sugar is one of the best ways to fight against diabetes. But there are several key nutrients that should be included in your diet to ensure complete recovery from type 2 diabetes.[44]

Nutrition Specifics in the Reversal of Type 2 Diabetes

There are several nutrients that are key to the fight against type 2 diabetes. Vitamins, minerals and phytonutrients all play their own roles, and we will go over them in detail here.

While there are many nutrients that are essential to human health, there are some in particular that someone with diabetes should make sure they are getting enough of:

- Chromium
- Vitamin D
- Vitamin C
- Beta-carotene
- Magnesium

Chromium

Chromium, for instance, has been an interest of studies for nutritional enhancement of glucose metabolism since the 1950s. These studies suggested that chromium was a critical cofactor in the action of insulin. In some studies, chromium has been found to impede phosphotyrosine phosphatase, the enzyme that severs phosphate from insulin receptors. This severing of phosphate from insulin receptors often leads to an increase in insulin resistance. The inhibition of phosphatase in conjunction with the activation of kinase (insulin's effector) would lead to increased phosphorylation of the receptor and an increase in insulin sensitivity. It has also been suggested that chromium increases insulin's receptor binding, the number of insulin receptors and beta cell sensitivity. Studies have also shown that insulin resistance and diabetes have been found to develop in animals and humans with low chromium levels.[56]

Chromium can be found in egg yolks, nuts, green beans, broccoli, brewer's yeast and meat. Low chromium levels are associated with a heavy intake of processed foods, refined grains and sugars. In addition to being very low in nutritive value and containing very little if any chromium, these types of food actually increase chromium's exportation from the body.[56]

Vitamin D

Vitamin D is another nutrient that has been found to have a role in the development of type 2 diabetes Preeti Kishore, MB, BS, an assistant professor at the Albert Einstein College of Medicine in New York, has done research on macrophages and the effect that vitamin D has on them. There is reason to believe that macrophages, a specialized immune system cell, are also something of a waste disposal cell as well. When fat cells get too large, they die – and researchers now believe that macrophages are in charge of cleaning up the dead cells. The heightened presence of macrophages in obese people's adipose tissue may be due to higher levels of cell death in their tissues and may contribute to the inflammation commonly associated with obesity.

Kishore's research on the macrophages has suggested that vitamin D deficiency causes the macrophages to become more active, and further contribute to insulin resistance and inflammation. As part of the study, Kishore gave eight people vitamin D supplements daily for two months. At the end of the study, the participants' hepatic insulin sensitivity, or liver insulin sensitivity, was up by nearly 37%. A lot of conventional scientists, especially those with pharmaceutical leanings, tend to feel that most evidence of vitamin D's positive effects on type 2 diabetes is purely circumstantial. Hopefully the findings of this study will be the beginning of change in the scientific community, and their views on nutrition.[57]

Another, more recent study led by Dr. Esther Krug, an assistant professor at Johns Hopkins University and endocrinologist at Sinai Hospital in Baltimore, MD, found that an astonishing number of diabetes patients were also suffering from a lack of vitamin D. The researchers also noted that the patients with higher A1C levels also had some of the lowest vitamin D levels, which points to the suggestion that vitamin D is an important player in long-term blood glucose control.[10]

Your skin produces vitamin D when it's exposed to sunlight. Experts say that the skin can produce enough of the vitamin in about 30 minutes of sun exposure. This time length varies upon several factors, such as how much skin is being exposed and what time and season it is. For example, laying out with your hands and face exposed at dusk is not going to yield the same amount of vitamin D production as laying out in your swimsuit at noon on a summer day. It can also be especially difficult to get enough vitamin D in the winter or if you live in a low-sunlight region. The recommended daily intake (RDI) for vitamin D is about 600 IU (international Units). Fortunately, there are some great food sources of vitamin D that can help one meet that need, and you can read more about supplementation in Chapter 6.

Fatty fish, such as salmon, trout and swordfish contain between 86 and 97% of the RDI for vitamin D per three-ounce serving. White fish and mackerel contain about 50%. Other fish such as tuna, halibut, sole and flounder are also excellent sources of vitamin D, though they may not pack as much punch per serving as salmon or swordfish. It is also important to make sure your fish is sourced ethically and carefully. Fish from the Pacific Ocean tend to be more contaminated than fish from the Atlantic. Sustainably farmed fish are also going to contain fewer toxins than those that are not sustain-ably farmed.

Mushrooms are a great vegetarian source of vitamin D as well, with some varieties containing up to 131% of the RDI. Other sources, such as beef, eggs, and tofu do exist, but they do not contain large enough quantities to be feasible sources on their own. [58]

Vitamin C

The antioxidant vitamin C may be quite beneficial for type 2 diabetic pa-tients. Studies have shown that low levels of vitamin C may be related to the onset of type 2 diabetes. Vitamin C has also been proven to help improve the processing of insulin and glucose in the body.[59]

A study conducted by the Institute of Metabolic Science at Addenbrooke's Hospital, Cambridge, England, that was published in the *Archives of Internal Medicine* also found that vitamin C is a great preventative. The study began with 21,831 healthy men and women having their blood vitamin C levels measured. Twelve years later, 3.2% of the study's population had developed type 2 diabetes. Upon evaluating the vitamin C levels in the subjects' blood along with their diabetes risk, the researchers found surprising results. Those with the highest vitamin C levels had a 62% lower risk of developing type 2 diabetes than those who had the lowest vitamin C levels.

The researchers also noted that vitamin C levels are a reliable measure of fruit and vegetable intake, and that the evidence is very supportive of the beneficial effects of vitamin C consumption along with fruit and vegetable consumption for the prevention of type 2 diabetes.[60]

Oranges are widely known as being the top choice for getting the daily dose of vitamin C, but there are plenty of other options out there to meet the suggested intake of 90 mg for men and 75 mg for women. Strawberries are an excellent alternative to oranges, as are papayas. Papaya is also rich in folate, an important B vitamin. A small papaya contains about 96 mg of vitamin C. Strawberries are a great low-calorie fruit and contain about 87 mg per serving. Both are excellent sources of fiber for fruit as well. Broccoli is one of the most popular green vegetables, and it also just so happen to be great sources of vitamin C too. Broccoli contains about 132 mg of vitamin C per serving, making it one of the richest sources for the nutrient. Cauliflower contains about 128 mg per serving and is also an excellent anti-inflammatory food.[61]

Beta-Carotene

Beta-carotene, the antioxidant found in much orange and red produce that's related to vitamin A, has also been shown to fight type 2 diabetes. A recent study concluded that the higher the intake of beta-carotene, the greater reduction there was in the risk for developing type 2 diabetes. Beta-carotene was proven to help protect against genetic risk factors for type 2 diabetes as well.[62]

The best sources of beta-carotene come from yellow, orange and red foods. Carrots, sweet potatoes, pumpkin, papaya and mango make up some of the best orange foods. Butternut squash, red bell peppers, apricots, cantaloupe and watermelons are some of the less conventional choices for meeting your beta-carotene needs. You may also be surprised to learn that bok choy, kale, collard greens and spinach are good sources of the nutrient as well, despite being green vegetables. The foods rich in beta-carotene are extremely healthy food choices, because in addition to this valuable nutrient, they are rich in fiber and many other key vitamins and minerals.[63]

Magnesium

Magnesium is another key player in the treatment of type 2 diabetes. Magnesium is a mineral that is essential to many of the key functions and enzymatic actions in the body. In fact, it's needed for more than 300 biochemical reactions, helps maintain normal nerve and muscle function and supports your immune system. Perhaps most notably in relation to diabetes, magnesium helps regulate your blood glucose.

Researchers from Harvard University's Medical School and School of Public Health conducted a study on how magnesium affects the risk of developing type 2 diabetes. The study followed 85,060 women for 18 years and 42,872 men for 12 years. This was a very large-scale study, and the researchers noted that an inverse association between magnesium levels and the onset of type 2 diabetes was consistent for men and women. The higher a person's intake of magnesium was, the less likely they were to develop the condition. The researchers also noted that this inverse correlation held true throughout multivariate modes. They concluded that magnesium may be protective against type 2 diabetes, but that it is likely more beneficial in people who are deficient in magnesium.[65]

There are many options for magnesium-rich foods to include in your daily diet. Leafy greens such as spinach, Swiss chard, beet and turnip greens are excellent sources of magnesium, containing 31 to 156 mg per serving, with spinach being the greatest source. Seeds and nuts are another great option, containing magnesium along with some healthy protein and fat. Pumpkin seeds contain about 192 mg of magnesium per one-ounce serving. Cashews provide 172 mg, and the ever-popular almond carries about 62 mg per quarter cup serving. Organic tempeh and tofu can also be great sources of magnesium, weighing in at 87 mg and 66 mg respectively.

Magnesium is also well known for being found in everyone's favorite treat, chocolate. Cacao contains a whopping 100 mg of magnesium per ounce, and cacao beans also boast some excellent antioxidant power. Dark chocolate is much higher in cacao and all of its health benefits than milk chocolate. Some other notable sources of food for magnesium are quinoa, summer squash, raspberries, black beans and seafood. The best way to get magnesium is through plants, as they generally contain the highest amounts of the nutrient.[66]

You can learn more about magnesium in the form of supplements in Chapter 6.

A Healthy Diet Paves the Way

Following a healthy diet is imperative to the reversal of type 2 diabetes. A healthy diet consists of whole, fresh foods that are rich in valuable vitamins and minerals. Vitamins and minerals are key to keeping your body functioning at its best, and to repairing the damage caused by processed foods, added sugars and trans fats. The hallmarks of the American diet do nothing but drag your body and your health through the mud.[44]

There are many toxic foods and food additives available at every corner store and supermarket, but that doesn't mean it's what you have to eat. Committing to a healthier, better way of eating will impact your life in many positive ways. Not only does eating a healthier diet help you manage your diabetes, but it will help you feel more motivated to be active, give you more energy, and reduce your risk for many other health issues and conditions, like heart disease. Following a healthy diet doesn't just give you control over diabetes, it gives you control of your life.

Diet is just the first step in recovering from type 2 diabetes. While it is of utmost importance, diet alone may not be enough to fully reverse your diagnosis. Lifestyle changes can help you beat type 2 diabetes and lead a healthier existence overall.

Know what to eat to protect yourself against diabetes

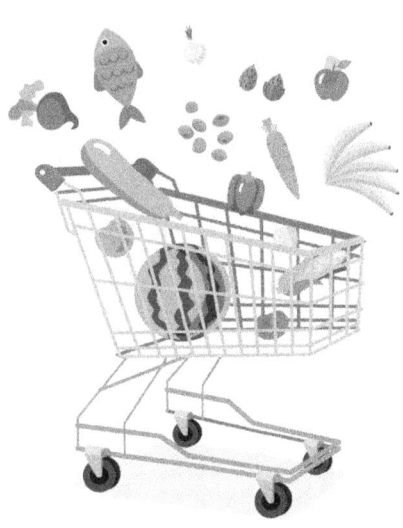 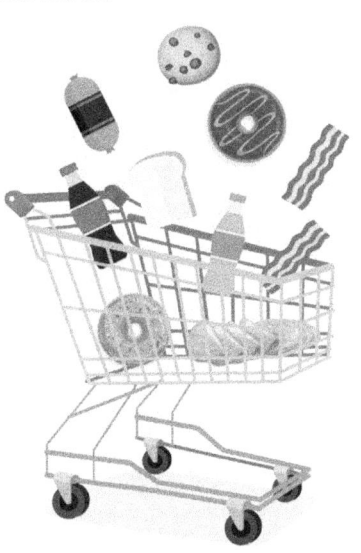

Consume:

- Fatty fish
- Fruits
- Vegetables
- Nuts/seeds
- Beans/legumes
- Whey protein

Avoid:

- Soda
- Sweets
- Refined grains
- Processed meats

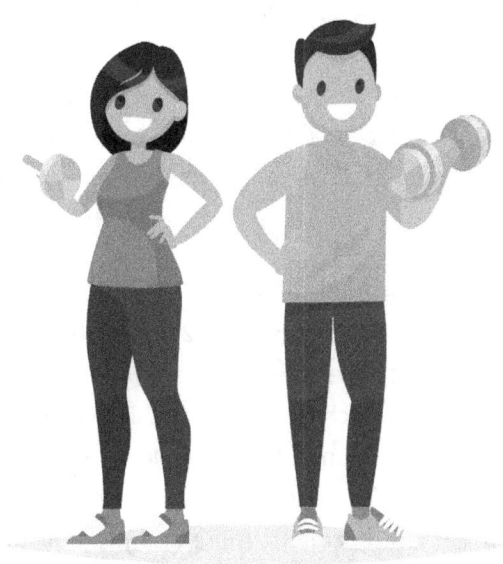

Chapter 5 – Lifestyle Changes to Reverse Diabetes

Changing your way of life is another prerequisite to overcoming diabetes. A certain lifestyle is associated with the development of type 2 diabetes and related complications. The fact is that being sedentary and following a poor diet, maybe even smoking, is not just a stereotype of the typical type 2 diabetic. These are proven risk factors in the progression of the disease.

There are many aspects to the Western lifestyle that contribute to the onset of type 2 diabetes, as well as other diseases and conditions. A sedentary lifestyle increases not only the risk of developing diabetes, but also your overall mortality risk. Most people in today's industrialized world do not have active lives. Sitting at a desk all day, going home, watching television until you fall asleep and repeating that routine day after day does nothing but kill you slowly. Worse yet, most people eat a bag of chips or some other snack food while they sit and do nothing. Mindless eating and mindless inactivity tend to go hand in hand. The worst thing you can ever do to yourself is fail to move. In our society, a lack of physical activity is far too common, and people are paying the price. Many conditions, like type 2 diabetes, can be prevented with regular exercise. Physical activity can also help reverse the condition as well.[67]

A 2013 study conducted by Bupa, a British insurance company, found that a quarter of British young adults, ages 18 to 24, walked 5 minutes or less per day. Can you imagine that? That seems to be on par with only getting up to walk to the bathroom, the kitchen and the car. The average isn't much better, either. The average woman in Britain walks about 12 minutes per day, while the average man walks only 8 minutes. It's no wonder that younger people, ages 25 to 30, are becoming more and more likely to develop diseases like type 2 diabetes.[68]

Though exercise is often thought of as just a way to lose weight, many studies have shown that the addition of exercise is one of the greatest ways to help reverse type 2 diabetes. A study published in *Archives of Internal Medicine* found that exercise and dietary intervention was more effective than medication at reversing the effects of type 2 diabetes.[38]

Exercise Provides Blood Sugar Benefits

Another study has also concluded that exercise in and of itself can improve blood glucose levels. A systematic review co-authored by Dr. Elizabeth Elliot of the University of Sydney and the Children's Hospital at Westmead in Australia found that, in addition to promoting healthy blood glucose levels, it also increases insulin sensitivity and decreases blood lipids. The study reviewed the findings of 14 randomized trials, featuring a total of 377 participants, with ages ranging from 45 to 65. All participants had type 2 diabetes. In the trials, subjects were randomly assigned to either partake in an exercise regime or not exercise. The types of exercise in each of the 14 trials varied, though different types of aerobic or resistance training were the most common. Participants in the exercise group had a 0.6% decrease in their A1C levels.[69]

The American Diabetes Association considers A1C values, or glycated hemoglobin values, the best way to monitor blood glucose levels. Though that may seem like a drop in the bucket, this represents a 30% improvement towards the goal of attaining an A1C value of 7% and a 20% improvement towards reaching a normal A1C lab value. In a press release announcing the study, Dr. Elliot said, "It's comparable to the drop that clinicians would like to see if prescribing medication."[69]

Patients in the exercise group also experienced a significant drop in triglycerides circulating in their bloodstream. Triglycerides tend to be higher in diabetic patients. The exercising test subjects also had a decrease in subcutaneous fat, as well as visceral fat, which is fat located around organs in the abdomen.[69]

Your body stores glucose in the form of glycogen. Glycogen is primarily found in the liver and in muscle tissue. When you exercise, your muscles use their glycogen stores. More glucose is used by muscle than other tissues. Active muscle tissue will burn up its glycogen stores. This allows the cells within the muscle tissue to absorb new glucose from the bloodstream and create new glycogen stores. This cycle of using up glycogen and refilling the stores promotes balanced blood sugar levels. Studies also show that muscle tissue is more sensitive to insulin and responds better after exercise. This serves to also help reverse insulin resistance and lower blood glucose levels.

Exercise also helps muscles more readily absorb glucose without as much need for insulin.[9] When you overeat and are inactive, it means you probably aren't burning through the glycogen that's already been stored away, and you are forcing your body to find something to do with all of the excess. Eventually, this cycle leads to weight gain and insulin resistance.[31]

Resistance Training Can Help

Resistance training, in particular, has recently been shown to also help prevent type 2 diabetes. It has been accepted for some time that aerobic exercise is beneficial to managing blood glucose, and a recent study published by *PLOS Medicine* shows that anaerobic activity may be just as important in reducing diabetes risk.

The study, which was carried out by researchers from Harvard University in conjunction with the University of Southern Denmark, suggests that strength training and conditioning can be equally preventative. The study utilized data from over 99,000 women that were middle-aged or older and had taken part in the Nurses' Health Study or the Nurses' Health Study II. None of the women had type 2 diabetes at the beginning of the study. The researchers analyzed their exercise habits and looked at frequency, duration and what type of exercise was being performed.

The researchers wanted to see what kind of relationship there was between their exercise routines and the occurrence of type 2 diabetes. Both resistance training, such as weight lifting, and lower-intensity muscle conditioning exercises like yoga were found to be independently successful at reducing diabetes risk. When combined, the two types of exercise were even more effective. The researchers noted that adding strength training and conditioning exercises in conjunction with aerobic exercise according to the current recommendation of physical activity provides substantial reduction in risk for developing type 2 diabetes in women.[70]

What are the recommended levels of activity? 150 minutes per week of aerobic activity and two sessions of resistance training or conditioning. Per the researchers' estimates, this should be at least 60 minutes total of strength and conditioning. Women who met these goals had the lowest risk of developing type 2 diabetes, but those who did not meet these specific amounts still had a reduction in risk.[70]

Men can also benefit from resistance training, of course. A study conducted by researchers from the same two institutions was published by the journal *Archives of Internal Medicine* in August of 2012. This research found that men reduced their risk of developing type 2 diabetes by 34% when they performed strength training regularly, or for about 30 minutes five times a week. It was also found that adding aerobic exercise such as running or walking promised even greater outcomes. Those who participated in regular aerobic activity in addition to anaerobic exercise saw a 59% decrease in their risk for developing type 2 diabetes. The most notable take-away from this is that both types of exercise provide a reduction in risk for diabetes independently. For people who may be unable to perform a specific activity due to injury, there are potential alternatives than can still be effective.[70]

Finding the time to exercise is one of the most important changes you can make in your life, in addition to changing the way you eat. Diet and fitness go hand in hand. If you are going to make the effort to change the way you eat, you should also make the effort to move more. You don't have to be perfect, but you do have to make some kind of effort to get results. If you want to reverse your type 2 diabetes, you're going to have to make time to exercise. Even if you start with 10 or 15 minutes a day, it's still better than nothing. You'll be surprised how quickly those minutes go by once you get used to doing it. Once you get your foot in the door, finding the time to eat well and get active will be like second nature.

Tobacco and Alcohol

Using tobacco is another lifestyle hurdle that must be overcome in order to beat type 2 diabetes. Smokers who smoke one pack or more per day actually double their risk of developing diabetes compared to non-smokers.[11] On average, smokers are at a 30 to 40% increased risk of developing type 2 diabetes. People that have diabetes and also smoke greatly increase their risk for developing severe complications related to their disease and their habit. For instance, smokers with diabetes are more likely to have poor blood flow. This poor blood flow can lead to infections that don't heal, ulcers and eventual amputation of the limbs – most commonly toes and feet. Diabetic smokers are also more likely to develop peripheral nerve damage and develop retinopathy, or damage to their retinas. They are also more likely to have trouble controlling their blood sugar levels, which worsens their condition and contributes to the development of those types of complications.[71]

Smoking cigarettes is associated with increased insulin resistance. This can lead to higher blood sugar levels, and the eventual development of type 2 diabetes. Smoking is unhealthy for your entire body. Though it may be difficult, the best thing you can do for yourself is quit. [72] If you are a smoker who wants to get healthy, quitting should be your top priority.

Consumption of alcohol can also impede your ability to manage your blood glucose levels if you are a type 2 diabetic. Alcohol has negative affects on your liver and the way it processes fat from the blood. This can in turn lead to increased risk of diabetic complications in conjunction with poor blood glucose control. [72]

Some studies do show that moderate alcohol consumption can be beneficial and reduce the risk of developing diabetes. However, moderation is the key. Moderate drinking is considered to be one drink per day for women of any age and for men over 65. Men under 65 years of age may consume up two drinks per day. Heavy drinking is associated with an increased risk in the development of type 2 diabetes.

Alcohol abuse can lead to pancreatitis, or inflammation of the pancreas. This inflammation can damage the organ's ability to secrete insulin effectively, which then leads to diabetes. [12] If you are already a diabetic, it is probably best to avoid drinking.

Antidepressants and Depression

Antidepressants have also been associated with type 2 diabetes. The exact correlation between the two remains unconfirmed. One study confirmed that patients that were taking two types of antidepressants, tricyclic antidepressants and selective serotonin re-uptake inhibitors, to manage their depression, had twice the risk of developing diabetes.

Researchers from the University of Southampton have conducted a meta-analysis of 22 studies on the subject of antidepressants and type 2 diabetes. They say that the use of antidepressants has soared dramatically in the last several years and that they are concerned that these drugs could be having a negative affect on consumers' glucose metabolism. The researchers noted that, in the United Kingdom, 46.7 billion people had prescriptions for antidepressants in 2011.[73]

In the United States, another study found that antidepressant drugs were the third most commonly prescribed medication. The team also found a general link between the long-term consumption of antidepressants and an increased risk of having poor blood glucose control. While they have also noted that study quality varied, all the most recent and larger studies suggest there is a correlation. While correlation does not equal causation, it certainly raises concerns about antidepressants.[73]

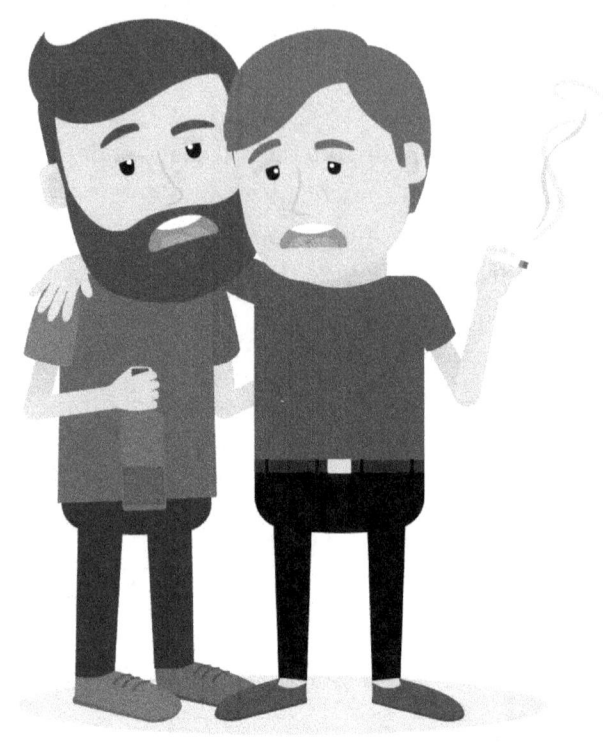

I don't know why I don't feel healthy.

In the United States, another study found that antidepressant drugs were the third most commonly prescribed medication. The team also found a general link between the long-term consumption of antidepressants and an increased risk of having poor blood glucose control. While they have also noted that study quality varied, all the most recent and larger studies suggest there is a correlation. While correlation does not equal causation, it certainly raises concerns about antidepressants. [73]

Dr. Katharine Barnard, who led the team, stated, "Our research shows that when you take away all the classic risk factors of type 2 diabetes; weight gain, lifestyle etc, there is something about antidepressants that appears to be an independent risk factor." She also noted that the potential risk is "quite worrying." Barnard also suggests that patients taking antidepressants need to be made aware of their heightened risk for developing type 2 diabetes while taking the medication.[73]

The majority has indeed become a mindless society. Today, people are unquestioningly taking pills to feel "better," or rather to feel nothing at all. It is much easier to take a drug than it is to actively correct what ails you. It requires no personal effort or betterment. The medication "fixes" the symptom, but never the problem. What is truly sad that the same things that cause diabetes – poor nutrition and lack of physical activity – bring about many cases of depression.

In fact, a study published in *Public Health Nutrition* found that people who frequently ate fast food and commercial baked goods like croissants and donuts increased their risk of developing depression by a whopping 51% compared to people who ate little or none of those foods. The study also found that people who ate larger quantities of these types of foods were more likely to be physically inactive and have a very poor diet. Typically, they were less likely to consume fruits, vegetables and healthy fats. The research also suggested that a high consumption of processed trans fats may interfere with the normal function of neurotransmitters in the brain, and disrupt the proper electrical activity essential for intercellular communication.[74]

It is also important to note that, if you are consuming a lot of unhealthy food, you probably aren't consuming enough nutrients to support a healthy, functioning body, and that includes your brain. For example, vitamin D and omega-3 fatty acids are considered essential to proper brain function, as are B vitamins. Elimination of refined sugars is also associated with relieving depression.[75] Isn't it amazing how these suggestions coincide with the dietary recommendations to reverse type 2 diabetes? Food is truly nature's best medicine if you are eating the right stuff. Though it can be difficult to find the motivation to improve your eating habits if you suffer from depression, it is truly a worthwhile endeavor.

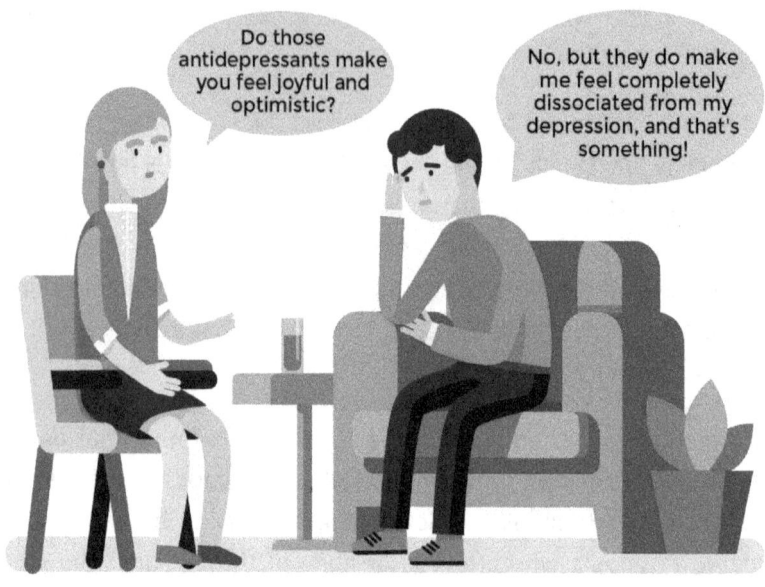

If you are taking a prescription medication for depression, you may want to voice concerns about the medication and your potential risks, but do not ever abruptly stop taking a medication without consulting with your doctor – many medications can have severe side affects with their cessation. Your doctor can help you step down off of a medication if that is what you wish to do. However, you can still start eating better to begin the healing process.

Depression is not a lifestyle choice, but your lifestyle choices can worsen the condition – making you more dependent on prescription drugs to correct the symptoms, just like type 2 diabetes. Getting your nutrition status on track can make a world of difference not just in your type 2 diabetes, but in terms of your mood and mental health as well.

Beliefs about Obesity and Lifestyle Changes

Being overweight is another key factor in the development of diabetes. Though not exactly a lifestyle, beliefs about your weight or size can still have dramatic impacts on your health. The "fat but fit" mentality does not exempt an overweight or obese individual from the fact that, regardless of their fitness level, they are still at an increased risk of mortality.

A recent study published in the *International Journal of Epidemiology* concluded that overweight people who where in the top tier of physical fitness still had a higher risk of death and disease than thin people, regardless of the thin person's fitness.[36] Being overweight is something of a lifestyle choice; you are choosing to either overeat or not exercise enough. If you are eating correctly, you should not be gaining weight unless you are seeking to gain muscle mass, or need to gain weight for other health reasons. If you are overweight, you should be eating to lose weight.

There is a mentality, especially among younger people, that being fat is okay. It is true that there are different body types, and some men and women are going to be larger than others. But there is a limit to what you can consider "body type" and what is really self-inflicted. A 60" waist is not a body type. It's a problem. The mainstream media loves to spin feel-good stories about how obesity is genetic. People want to believe there's nothing they can do about being overweight, so they have an excuse to be complacent in their lives.

Another popular "theory" is that obesity doesn't cause health problems. This is not based in reality, and is certainly not based on scientific evidence. A proponent of this movement, also called "Health At Every Size" is Dr. Linda Bacon. Dr. Bacon has written a popular book titled *Health At Every Size* in support of the movement. On the surface, it doesn't seem so bad. Everyone should take part in healthy lifestyle changes, regardless of their present weight.

Dr. Bacon says on the rear cover of her book to "find the joy in movement," which is a fairly benign suggestion. However, she also suggests, "Eat what you want, when you want, choosing pleasurable foods that help you feel good."[76] Now that suggestion is definitely more harmful than benign. Countless studies have proven that what you eat and what you weigh does in fact affect your risk for disease and mortality.[21]

In addition to the recently published study mentioned earlier which found that fat people had a higher risk for mortality than thin people, regardless of weight, many studies have found that eating more nutrient-rich foods, and less refined sugar, helps reduce depression.[75] Suggesting that people should eat only what feels pleasurable to them is ludicrous at best and dangerously irresponsible at worst.

Dr. Bacon also claims that her "plan" – if you can call it that – is "scientifically proven to improve health and self-esteem." Naturally, these claims are supported by her "government-funded academic studies." She proposes that the problem is not obesity, but rather that the problem is society. I suppose if you can convince yourself that it's okay to be fat, and it's not your fault that you're fat, you might very well have an increase in self-esteem. After all, you're not taking responsibility for yourself anymore.[76]

Dr. Bacon also has a chart on the back of her book listing a few "myths" and "realities" about being overweight. Her first "myth" is that "fat kills."[76] The research published in the *Journal of Epidemiology* proves her assertion to be incorrect.[36] And let's not forget the numerous studies that prove being overweight or obese increases your risk factors for numerous diseases and conditions, not the least of which are diabetes and diabetes-related disabilites.[21]

Dr. Bacon also claims that no study has ever proven that losing weight will help you live a longer life.[76] Again, the study on obesity and risk of mortality published in the *Journal of Epidemiology* suggests that being thinner does indeed increase your chances of living a longer life. It has also been proven by scientific studies that being overweight or obese increases the likelihood you will develop type 2 diabetes.[13] And, further research conducted by the CDC along with researchers from Emory University concluded that diabetes increases the number of years a person is likely to suffer from disability and shorten their lifespan.[21]

A study published in the *Annals of Internal Medicine* in 2015 which suggests that overweight diabetic patients live longer is often used to further the opinion that being fat is good. Where these people tend to get confused is whether the perceived benefit is from having extra weight or extra fat.

Dr. Carl Lavie, a cardiologist at the University of Queensland School of Medicine Ochsner Clinical School in New Orleans and a co-author of papers on the "obesity paradox" – what doctors have named the confounding evidence that being overweight may be protective – says that it's not body fat that's especially helpful. Dr. Lavie and his colleagues went on to analyze the lean index, or the amount of non-adipose tissue, in 48,000 patients. What they found was that, at higher BMIs, fat does indeed increase your mortality risk. Having more muscle and bone mass is what seems to be protective.[77] This makes sense when you consider that prior studies indicated that the "obesity paradox" really only offered positive, life-prolonging effects to people who were above a BMI of 25, but below a BMI of 30.[78]

Perhaps the most blasphemous assertion that Dr. Bacon makes is that, after reading her book, "you will be convinced the best way to win the war against fat is to give up the fight."[76] That alone tells you all you really need to know, doesn't it? Life is obviously much easier when someone encourages you to believe that giving up is actually better for you than pushing yourself.

Dr. Bacon is not the only person to suggest that eating whatever you want, whenever you want just because it "feels good" is the path to "health." Other books, such as *Intuitive Eating* by Evelyn Tribole and Elyse Recsh, both registered dietitians, echo similar sentiments. Intuitive eating can work for some people – if they have a healthy relationship with food and primarily choose things their body actually needs, like fruits and vegetables. *Intuitive Eating* boasts across its rear cover that you can "rediscover the pleasure of eating"and be freed from the dieting mindset.[76] Empowering books encouraging you to eat as you please can be quite beneficial to an anorexic. But is that same book helpful to a type 2 diabetic who is obese? No. It's harmful to that person, because it is encouraging them to continue behaviors that make them sick.

In the book, they discuss Michael Phelps – the Olympian infamous, in part, for his 12,000-calorie-a-day diet. They discuss how Phelps often ate fried egg sandwiches with onions and mayo for breakfast, ham and cheese sandwiches and a pound of enriched pasta for lunch, and another pound of pasta with a large pizza for dinner.[79] This is not healthy for the average human, not just in quantity, but quality – and it is not a healthy long-term diet. Phelps is an elite athlete, and an elite endurance athlete at that. That is an enormous amount of carbohydrates, but he specifically ate that way to fuel his training.

Their point of discussing Phelps was to dismiss the idea that eating certain foods can make you unhealthy or healthy.[79] They are missing the point that Phelps needed to eat that much food in order to have the energy to perform his training each day. He was training for the Olympics! That kind of diet is not one he would follow year-round if he wasn't training. Also, have you ever tried to eat 12,000 calories in salads? When you have that kind of caloric need, you do tend to eat what is calorie-dense.

Despite being dietitians, Tribole and Recsh seem to misconstrue what is good for an Olympic athlete with massive calorie needs while in training as being relevant to the average person. For people who are at risk of developing chronic conditions, or already have them, these kinds of "eat what feels good" and "no food can make you unhealthy" mentalities can be detrimental to their long-term health. It may feel good to eat that double cheeseburger and fries now, but in five or ten years and a thousand burgers later, you won't be enjoying them anymore. Maybe you'll need to get a foot amputated, maybe you'll lose your eyesight. You might be in a hospital receiving dialysis treatment. If you think it's hard to eat healthy now, just wait until you're on a renal diet. So, do you think all the cheeseburgers are worth it?

Intuitive eating basically suggests that you can eat what you want, when you want, without any consequences.[79] It would be more rational to suggest that this is not a good idea for most people until they have their habits and cravings under control. Once you are eating a diet based around good, wholesome foods and have created a more active lifestyle, it is generally okay to eat what you want – because you have hopefully retrained your body to crave healthy foods. When you eat well, fast food and pastries will hardly ever cross your mind. Good food is so much more satisfying and nutritious. If you crave a nice big salad with some beans or lentils – by all means, eat that for lunch whenever you want! That is a healthy craving.

Intuitive eating, for the individual who is choosing healthy foods, can be beneficial. It suggests more mindful eating – being aware of when you are hungry and when you feel full.[79] Those things can be very helpful. Eating intuitively can be quite good for you, if you are able to do so healthfully.

Your beliefs about what you can and cannot do can be very limiting, if you let them. It is more important that you believe in yourself, and your ability to follow through with changing your life, than any single action you could take. If you don't believe you can actually do it, you never will. It doesn't matter what you weigh or what you eat if you aren't actively participating in your own life. To truly reverse type 2 diabetes, you need to acknowledge and accept responsibility for your life, your body and everything in between.

You don't have to be perfect. You just have to start making the effort. Start small and work your way up. It will get easier to be healthy. Once you start eating healthy food, you won't crave the junk anymore. Once you start walking, it will get easier to keep doing it. You might even find that you enjoy taking a brisk walk every day, and maybe you'll start to enjoy seeing yourself attaining your goals and surpassing them. Good nutrition and healthy habits aren't going to just reverse your type 2 diabetes. You'll find that they are also a great way to jump-start your zest for life.

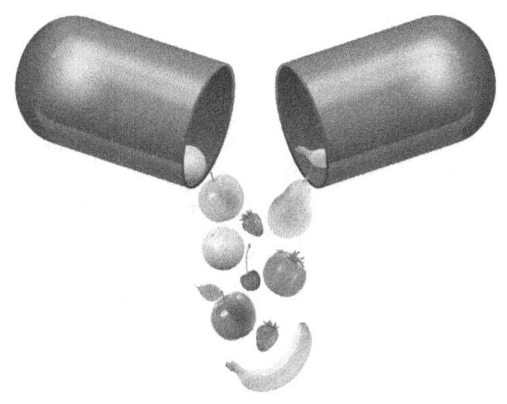

Chapter 6 – Supplements to Improve Your Health

Supplements are no replacement for a healthy diet and lifestyle. They can, however, support your efforts and help assist you with reaching your goals. Natural supplements can be used to enhance your health and improve your body's ability to control blood sugar levels on its own. Supplements can also help with other aspects of type 2 diabetes, such as high cholesterol and high triglycerides. There are many different types of supplements than can be taken, but you should always consult with your doctor before taking anything, especially if you are already on any type of medication or supplement to ensure there are no contraindications between supplements or special considerations that should be made.

For example, if you take an iron supplement and a vitamin C supplement, your doctor might suggest you take them together to increase absorption. Supplements can be very beneficial to your overall health and wellness. You will likely find yourself feeling better than you ever have as you continue along the journey of reversing type 2 diabetes. It is both motivating and satisfying to get healthy. So, what else can help you along the way?

Probiotics

Probiotics have recently been shown to do many great things for the body. One of these great things, according to a meta-analysis of several international studies conducted by researchers at the University of Science, Malaysia, found that healthy levels of gut bacteria and consumption of probiotics led to a reduction in insulin resistance significant enough to prevent the onset of type 2 diabetes.

Another study conducted in 2013 by researchers from Kashan, Iran, took 54 type 2 diabetics and split them into two groups, a probiotic group and a placebo group, and studied them for eight weeks. During these eight weeks, the probiotic group's fasting blood glucose levels were consistently lower than the placebo group. Although insulin resistance continued to increase in both groups of patients, the probiotics group experienced a much lower increase in insulin resistance than the placebo group. The probiotic group also had higher levels of antioxidants in their blood stream and lower levels of the arterial stress marker C-reactive protein.[80]

Probiotics can be taken in the form of a pill as a supplement, or you can eat probiotic foods. Fermented vegetables, like sauerkraut, are a delicious way to eat your vegetables and get a double whammy of nutritional benefits and probiotic benefits. If you prefer to go a little spicy, kimchi is a popular Korean fermented cabbage dish. Kefir is a popular fermented beverage that is most commonly compared to yogurt, but it can be made with water, grains or coconut water. Kombucha is a sweetened, tea-based drink that is also fermented. Apple cider vinegar is a health-food staple that is made from fermented apples. It contains probiotics and is also known for being quite helpful at stabilizing blood sugar levels.

Probiotic foods are essential for a healthy gut, strong immune system and improved digestion.[81] They can also be considered very beneficial for blood sugar stabilization and a reduction in heart disease risk.[80]

Cinnamon

Cinnamon is also a very valuable tool to the type 2 diabetic. Not only is it a wonderful, warming spice – it has very powerful antioxidant and blood sugar stabilizing capabilities. Cinnamon acts to balance blood glucose levels by stimulating insulin receptors. This increases their sensitivity to the hormone and lowers the amount of insulin needed to create the desired response. In return, the body doesn't need to produce as much insulin, and this lowers the amount of stress being placed on the pancreas, decreases inflammation and improves overall metabolism.

There are two different types of cinnamon, Ceylon cinnamon and cassia. Cassia is the more common variety, which you will often find in grocery stores. They are from the same family and provide many of the same benefits. Ceylon is considered to be the "true" and more medicinal form of cinnamon, since it contains higher amounts of antioxidant compounds. The real major difference between the two is coumarin content. Coumarin is a blood-thinning agent found in many different plants. Cassia cinnamon contains a much higher amount of coumarin than Ceylon, and should be used in moderation. It is nearly impossible to tell which type of cinnamon you have unless it's labeled and you're purchasing from a reputable source – so it's best to just stick to moderation.

One half teaspoon a day is more than enough to reap the great antioxidant and blood-sugar-stabilizing effects of cinnamon.[82] One easy way to add cinnamon to your diet is by adding a little bit to a smoothie or protein shake. You can also sprinkle a little cinnamon on sliced fruits such as apples, peaches or bananas for a healthy treat.

Supplements that can be beneficial include:

- Probiotics
- Cinnamon
- Spirulina
- Chlorella
- Aloe vera
- Green tea
- Ginger
- Turmeric
- Astaxanthin
- Fish oil
- Whey protein
- Chia seeds
- Silymarin
- Selenium
- Magnesium
- Vitamin D

Spirulina

Spirulina is another popular superfood known for its vast array of health benefits. A Korean study sought to find out if the benefits of spirulina extended to the treatment of type 2 diabetics, and they had some very positive findings. In the study, 37 diabetics were randomly assigned to be in the spirulina-receiving group or the control group. Both groups were required to maintain their usual diets without adding any other supplements or superfoods. Though spirulina supplementation did nothing to help the subjects decrease their BMIs, or body mass indexes, they did see significant decreases in serum triglyceride levels and blood pressure.

Type 2 diabetics frequently have high levels of triglycerides in their blood in addition to hypertension. Spirulina supplementation also significantly reduced malondialdehyde levels in the bloodstream, which is a biomarker for oxidative stress. The subjects receiving the superfood also experienced an increase in adiponectin levels, which is linked to increased insulin sensitivity and a decreased risk of heart attack. The researchers concluded that spirulina can be very beneficial to type 2 diabetics, especially in regard to improving blood lipid profiles and antioxidant capacity along with reducing inflammation.

One caveat to spirulina is that some strains of cyanobacteria, also known as blue-green algae, can actually be quite harmful to the body, and toxic to the liver. It is important to purchase wisely and carefully from a reputable manufacturer with stringent quality control practices.[83]

Chlorella

If spirulina seems a little too risky, but you would like to get the benefits of algae, look no further than chlorella – which has not currently been shown to have those same potential downsides.[83] Chlorella is a single-cell microalga and a multifaceted superfood. To complete its repertoire of heightening immune function, boosting liver health and fighting cancer, it seems only natural that this little powerhouse can help reverse diabetes too. Several studies have concluded that chlorella consumption can help manage blood sugar levels.

The first study, conducted in South Korea in 2009, conducted with diabetic and healthy rats, found that the consumption of chlorella was able to create a hypoglycemic effect that balanced out the hyperglycemia associated with insulin resistance – without pushing the pancreas to secrete more insulin. Another study conducted in Taiwan concluded that chlorella effectively has the ability to lower insulin resistance and improve insulin sensitivity and that it may be used as an adjuvant therapy. Both of these studies exhibit potential for chlorella to help reverse high blood sugar levels and insulin resistance in type 2 diabetics. [84]

Aloe Vera

Another great superfood for the type 2 diabetic is *Aloe vera*. *Aloe vera* is more than just a pretty plant; it is one of nature's best medicines. The gel found within the leaves of the *Aloe vera* plant is extremely healing for many internal and external conditions. *Aloe vera* has many uses because of this. It is commonly used to treat sunburns and other types of wounds because of its calming and soothing nature, but it can do far more. When consumed, *Aloe vera* gel can help reduce inflammation throughout the body – which is a common symptom of type 2 diabetes. Inflammation related to being overweight is also thought to be a proponent in the onset of the disease as well. *Aloe vera* also stabilizes blood sugar levels.

Diabetics who have consistently consumed the plant's gel for three months have been shown to experience a significant drop in fasting blood glucose levels. Studies also show that consuming *Aloe vera* reduces cholesterol and triglycerides in the bloodstream, and re-balances blood chemistry. Type 2 diabetics are at an increased risk of developing high cholesterol and high triglycerides due to the nature of their condition. This super-healing plant has also been shown to improve circulation to the extremities – another very important thing for type 2 diabetics to protect against peripheral neuropathy.

One of the best things about *Aloe vera* is that the gel is totally safe to eat. It's a medicinal food, and its not toxic like the many drugs you may be prescribed to treat all the aspects of diabetes. In conventional medicine, you need a drug to treat the elevated blood sugars, a drug for the cholesterol and a drug for the high triglycerides. And then they probably have to give you something else to treat all the side effects! It's insane, especially when you realize that the only medicine you need can be provided by nature.[85]

Green Tea

Green tea is also a great choice to add to your day, particularly if you start drinking unsweetened green tea to replace soda! Not only is it an excellent replacement for the unhealthy, high-fructose corn syrup-laden beverage of America, but it's got an astounding array of health benefits to boot.

One of green tea's many medicinal compounds, epigallocatechin gallate, or EGCG, has been shown to improve glucose tolerance in diabetic rodents, according to a study conducted by DSM Nutritional Products. The study divided 41 diabetic mice into five groups: two control groups that received either a placebo or a diabetic drug and three groups that received varying amounts of EGCG. All of the mice receiving EGCG experienced vast improvements in blood glucose levels at the five-week mark.

The group being given the highest amount (10 grams) experienced an improvement in blood sugar of nearly 50%. At six weeks, all of the rats receiving EGCG also showed improved levels of free fatty acids in their blood along with continued betterment of blood glucose levels and insulin tolerance. The level of improvement in the rats proved to be dose-dependent, but even those on the smallest amount of EGCG still experienced noticeable changes. The researchers concluded that EGCG could potentially be quite beneficial to humans with type 2 diabetes as well.[86]

The catechins in green tea have other benefits as well, such as promoting a reduction in abdominal fat – one of the risk factors in the development and progression of type 2 diabetes. Drinking four to five cups of green tea daily along with regular exercise has been proven to bolster weight loss efforts and help reduce central adiposity. Green tea is also thought to contain thermogenic properties that help your body use its energy stores more effectively throughout the day. A few other benefits to green tea include its antioxidant powers, which help reduce oxidative stress, lower blood pressure and preserve healthy cholesterol levels. These qualities are all extremely beneficial to a type 2 diabetic.

Type 2 diabetes is associated with an increase in oxidative stress in the body, along with elevated LDL cholesterol and high blood pressure. The disease is cyclical in that these symptoms play off each other, each making the other worse. The compounds in green tea can help reduce these symptoms, and there is nothing more relaxing than a cup of green tea.[87]

Ginger

Ginger is another potential option in reversing type 2 diabetes. A study published in the *International Journal of Food Sciences and Nutrition* found that ginger was effective at increasing insulin sensitivity. The study was a randomized, double-blind study in which people were assigned to take either a placebo or 2 g of ginger daily for two months. At the end of the study, researchers found that the subjects taking ginger had significantly better insulin sensitivity, lower levels of LDL (bad) cholesterol and lower levels of triglycerides.

The findings of another study, published in 2012 by researchers from the University of Sydney, suggested that ginger extract helped increase cellular uptake of glucose independent of insulin. More specifically, the compounds in ginger extract, special polyphenols called "gingerols," were found to promote the distribution of GLUT4.[88] You may recall GLUT4 from Chapter 1. GLUT4 is the glucose transporter found in insulin-responsive tissues such as skeletal muscle and adipose tissue. Insulin is the primary stimulator for the release of glucose transporters such as GLUT4.[6] It is quite impressive to see that gingerols are able to encourage an increase in GLUT4 independent of insulin.

Ginger has many other benefits and is one of the most commonly used medicinal herbs in the world. It can help treat harmful inflammation, which can also be beneficial for type 2 diabetics.[88]

Turmeric

Turmeric is another popular health-promoting herb; it is often used in curries but is now being recognized for its many medicinal uses. A study led by Dr. Drew Tortoriello, an endocrinologist and research scientist at the Naomi Berrie Diabetes Center at Columbia University Medical Center focused on determining whether turmeric would be beneficial in preventing diabetes in obese mice. Dr. Tortoriello and his colleagues learned that turmeric-fed mice had a much lower chance of developing type 2 diabetes, based on blood sugar levels, along with glucose and insulin tolerance tests. The turmeric-fed mice also had much lower levels of inflammation in their tissues and liver. The researchers hypothesize that curcumin, the anti-inflammatory antioxidant compound in turmeric, may be protective against insulin resistance and type 2 diabetes by lessening the inflammatory response promoted by obesity.[89]

Astaxanthin

Astaxanthin is another type of antioxidant produced by algae, yeast and sea life that has anti-inflammatory properties and a vast array of other health benefits. Astaxanthin is truly a miracle from Mother Nature for the type 2 diabetic, as it can help lower blood sugar levels as well as prevent damage from the disease. For example, type 2 diabetics frequently suffer kidney damage. Astaxanthin can help protect kidneys from damage, and reduce the chances of developing diabetic kidney disease. Astaxanthin has also shown it has the capacity to stabilize blood sugar levels, which in turn helps prevent the advancement of type 2 diabetes and the progression of its complications.

Astaxanthin can also improve your cardiovascular health, workout performance and muscle recovery. This can be beneficial to type 2 diabetics seeking to increase their activity levels for several reasons. The first and foremost might be that, with increased recovery and greater strides in cardiovascular health improvements, it might help keep new exercisers' motivation high and help keep you from getting too discouraged. If you're feeling great, you'll want to keep feeling that way. Astaxanthin may also help you feel better about the effort you are putting into exercising given that it has been shown to help improve performance during workouts and overall endurance.

Astaxanthin may also help protect your body from damage caused by oxidative stress, which is considered an instigator in the progression of type 2 diabetes. Astaxanthin is also a fat-soluble phytonutrient, making it rather unique. This is in large part why it is so very beneficial, and why it is able to help produce so many positive effects, like better blood glucose control and advanced muscle recovery. By being stored in the tissues instead of just circulating through the bloodstream and out again, like water-soluble nutrients do, astaxanthin is better able to protect your cells from degeneration and oxidation. For the type 2 diabetic, this is extremely important to protect against further damage to fragile blood vessels, nerves and kidneys and prevent advanced complications of the disease. Astaxanthin can also help stabilize blood sugar levels, which is imperative to the reversal of type 2 diabetes.[90]

Fish Oil

Fish oil is another supplement you may consider taking, to help boost your omega-3 fatty acid intake. A 2013 study published in the *Journal of Clinical Endocrinology & Metabolism* suggests that a regular intake of fish oil supplements may help prevent and reduce diabetes risk. The researchers posit that this is because fish oil increases adiponectin, a hormone found in human blood. Higher levels of adiponectin are also associated with a reduction in heart disease risk. The hormone is also linked to regulation of glucose metabolism and inflammation. At the study's conclusion, the results were unclear as to whether fish oil supplementation actually affected glucose metabolism as it relates to type 2 diabetes. The results did however support earlier findings that fish oil supplementation helps control blood glucose metabolism and aids in the metabolism of fat cells.[91]

A 20-year study that began in the 1980s was more recently published in 2014 by the journal *Diabetes Care*. Researchers from the University of Eastern Finland conducted the study, which utilized data from 2,212 men. At the beginning of the study, the men had their serum omega-3 fatty acid levels measured. Four-day food recalls along with self-administered questionnaires and oral glucose tolerance blood tests were also performed. Throughout the study, the men were divided into four groups based on the amount of omega-3 fatty acids they consumed. At the study's conclusion, it was found that men who had the highest concentrations of omega-3 fatty acids had a 33% reduction in risk for developing type 2 diabetes.[92]

Whey Protein

Whey protein is another supplement you may consider taking. A recent study published in the *Journal of Proteome Research* and funded by the Nordic Centre of Excellence and the Danish Council for Strategic Research found that consuming whey protein yielded positive results for obese individuals. In the study, the researchers fed volunteers a meal supplemented with one of several types of protein. The volunteers who received whey protein had lower levels of fatty acids in their blood after the meal, as well as higher levels of amino acids, which are known to help promote better insulin levels. The findings suggest that whey protein supplementation could help lower the risk for type 2 diabetes.

Many other studies have found positive effects of whey protein supplementation on the body, such as one conducted by researchers at Washington State University that was published in the *International Dairy Journal* and found that taking a whey supplement helped reduce high blood pressure.[93]

Silymarin

Silymarin, an antioxidant-filled extract of milk thistle, is also thought to be quite beneficial to diabetics for a number of reasons. A study published in *Phytotherapy Research* looked at 51 patients over a period of two years. Twenty-five of the participants received a 200 mg supplement of silymarin three times a day for four months. The remaining participants received a placebo at the same frequency and duration. The group given silymarin showed significant reductions in glycated hemoglobin (A1C) levels and fasting blood glucose levels. The results suggest that silymarin may be beneficial for lowering blood glucose levels and stabilizing them. The flavolignans found in milk thistle have also been shown to help protect the liver from damage.[94]

Chia Seeds

Chia seeds have recently experienced a surge in popularity , and they also contain nutrients and antioxidants that can help reverse type 2 diabetes. A 2009 study published in the *British Journal of Nutrition* concluded that chia seed consumption can help reverse insulin resistance as well as lower the amount of lipids and cholesterol found in the bloodstream. The results of the study were attributed to the fact that chia seeds form a gel when consumed, which helps slow digestion and absorption of the sugars in carbohydrates. This allows the sugars to be broken down and absorbed slowly and steadily by the body, reducing the likelihood of blood glucose spikes.

Chia seeds are also packed with valuable nutrients and healthy fats. In fact, a once-ounce serving of chia seeds contains nearly 25% of the RDI for magnesium. Magnesium is one of the many important minerals for reversing type 2 diabetes. Chia seeds are also an excellent source of protein and fiber, which is another key aspect to treating the condition. Chia seeds also have a great omega fatty acid profile, with an optimal omega-3 to omega-6 ratio that is known to help improve brain function. Chia seeds host all the amazing benefits of omega-3 and omega-6 fatty acids, such as cancer prevention and lowering the risk of heart disease and diabetes.

Chia seeds are also said to be a great energy booster, perfect for the person seeking to add more exercise to their life. These wonderful little seeds are truly a nutrient powerhouse and have many benefits for type 2 diabetics seeking to reverse their condition. They can be eaten plain or added to smoothies, cereals or salads.[95]

Adding Micronutrient Supplements

Before beginning any supplementation, you should always consult with your naturopathic physician or doctor first, particularly if you are already taking any kind of supplement or medication. This is especially true if you are considering supplementing vitamins or minerals, especially those that are fat-soluble such as vitamin D. Fat-soluble vitamins and minerals are much more likely to cause toxicity if too much is consumed.

It is best to make sure you are in fact deficient in a vitamin or mineral before taking a supplement for it. It is also good to discuss any dietary changes you may wish to make with your physician or naturopath as well. If you are planning on increasing your dietary intake of specific nutrients, a professional can help guide you with what supplementation, if any, would be beneficial to you. For example, if you are vitamin D-deficient but you want to eat more fatty fish and mushrooms, your physician may have a different recommendation for you than someone who is vitamin D-deficient and allergic to fish or mushrooms.

Selenium

Selenium is a particularly controversial mineral in regard to the onset or prevention of type 2 diabetes. For example, a study published in the journal *Diabetes Care* concluded that high levels of the mineral can actually increase the prevalence of diabetes, while it has also been suggested that selenium could be beneficial for type 2 diabetes prevention, because of its antioxidant capacity and other benefits.[96]

Observational studies and randomized trials have reached both positive and negative findings. A 2012 study conducted by researchers from the University of Surrey in England concluded that selenium supplementation in individuals with relatively low selenium levels did not increase their diabetes risk.[97] So, if you are deficient in the mineral and your physician recommends taking a supplement for it, you should be just fine.

Magnesium

Magnesium supplements can be particularly difficult to navigate, because there are a number of different forms available on the market. Not all types of magnesium are created equal, however. Some of the worst forms of magnesium are magnesium oxide, magnesium sulfate, magnesium glutamate and magnesium aspartate.[98]

Magnesium oxide is considered an inferior source of magnesium due to its poor rate of absorption. Despite being the most common form sold in pharmacies, it's woefully inadequate because it's non-chelated. Magnesium sulfate, also known as Epsom salt, has many uses but is unsafe for supplementation purposes. Magnesium glutamate and magnesium aspartamate should be avoided completely, due to the neurotoxic nature of glutamic and aspartic acids.[98]

So what kinds of magnesium are good? Magnesium citrate is an excellent option, because it is affordable, readily available and easily absorbed. Magnesium glycinate and magnesium carbonate are other good alternatives that are absorbed well. Magnesium glycinate is one of the safest options and has the added benefit of being the least likely to cause diarrhea.[98]

There are a number of vitamins and minerals that are beneficial for the management of type 2 diabetes. It is always most beneficial to try to consume these nutrients through food. However, some nutrients can be difficult to get enough of, especially if you have special dietary considerations, such as food allergies or other dietary preferences. For example, a person who is vegan may have difficulty getting enough of all the B vitamins.

After discussing your dietary preferences with your doctor, and what methods of alternative therapy you are thinking about trying – together you can come up with a nutrition, exercise and supplement plan personally tailored to fit your needs.

Supplements have many benefits!

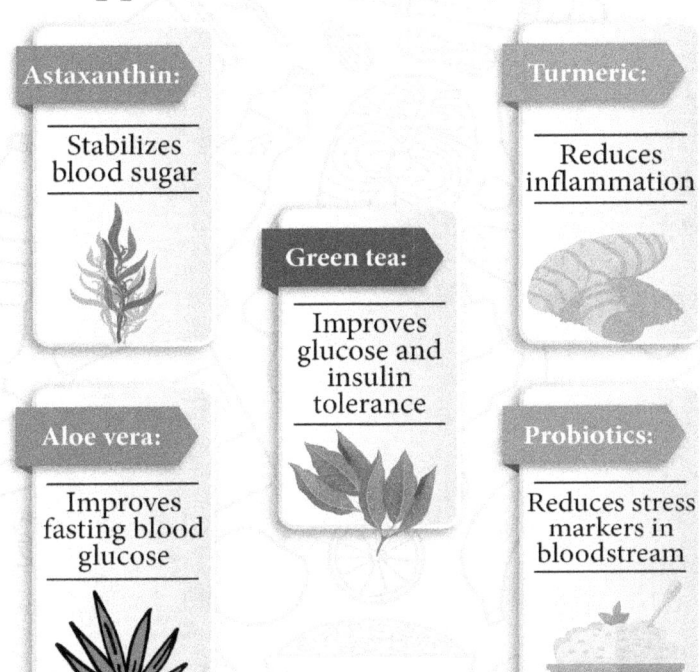

Astaxanthin:
Stabilizes blood sugar

Turmeric:
Reduces inflammation

Green tea:
Improves glucose and insulin tolerance

Aloe vera:
Improves fasting blood glucose

Probiotics:
Reduces stress markers in bloodstream

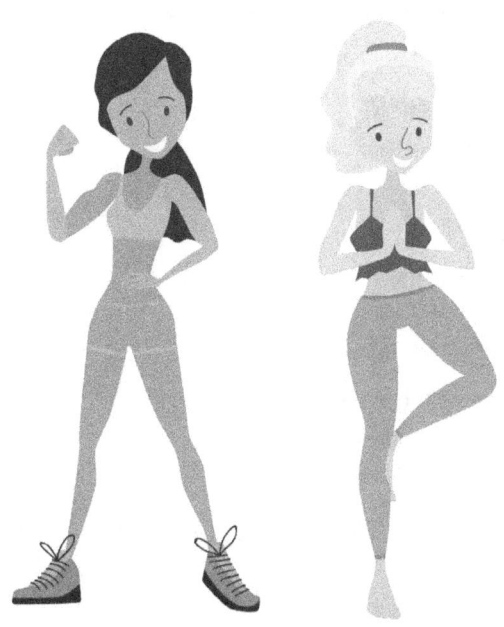

Conclusion

In order to overcome a disease like diabetes, one must also embark on a path to wellness. And as this book explains, health and wellness is not created by any one particular activity, supplement or food: it is created through a harmony of all those very things. These tools are able to provide you some benefits individually, of course, but when used together – the outcome will be many times greater.

By gaining a better understanding of what causes diabetes, you can rest assured knowing that it does not have to be a death sentence. Furthermore, by gaining an understanding of why conventional treatment may not be working for you, you have hopefully gaining a new sense of hope for the future, rife with the knowledge that you have the power to change the quality of your life and your health.

Things that contribute to or worsen type 2 diabetes:
- Lack of physical activity
- Being overweight or obsese
- Excess belly fat
- Poor eating habits
- Nutrient deficiencies
- Trans fats
- Added sugars and high-fructose corn syrup
- Refined grains and high-glycemic index foods
- Sugar-sweetened beverages
- Artificial sweeteners
- Certain types of medications, including diabetes drugs themselves
- Tobacco use
- Alcohol abuse

Making the changes necessary to overcome diabetes are not easy: to undergo a lasting change requires quite a lot of determination. But you also have to be understanding and patient with yourself. If you have a set back, one of the worst things you can do is throw in the towel. A defeatist attitude will not get you very far on the road to better health, and you won't get very far anywhere else in life, either.

As I said in the beginning, you alone have the power to change your health. By changing what you put into your system, you can change what you get out of it. There is perhaps nothing more empowering – nor more daunting – than accepting that you alone have that kind of power in your own life.

You do not need to be a pawn of the corrupt medical system. While the puppets of the pharmaceutical industry may like for you to believe that medication is the only thing that can help you gain control of your health, there is plenty of evidence to show that this is simply not the truth: there are other ways. Natural wellness is always an option, but you first have to choose it. No conventional doctor will tell you how to choose the right foods or how to supplement your diet. They may give you the trite platitudes about healthy eating we've all heard before, but the truth is, most of them don't know how to help you overcome a disease without giving you medication.

Better health is well within your reach, and one of the first places you can start is the kitchen. Ditch the junk food, the artificial ingredients and the sugar-laden snacks. Keep your kitchen clean, and by that I mean eat clean, wholesome foods that are nutrient-dense and free of nutritionally depleted additives and ingredients. Soon, you won't crave the junk food anymore, and you may even find that you don't even like it anymore.

The next step is working on your lifestyle. Exercise is key, but don't feel defeated if it's hard at first. Everything is hard when you first start out, and everything gets easier over time. Even if you just start with ten or fifteen minutes a day, that's a great way to begin a more active life. Eating well and engaging in physical activity are truly the corner stones of human health. Those two things alone can truly improve your life more than just about anything else, and without them, no other efforts you may choose to make will be quite as profound. Taking a dietary supplement while eating a junk food diet and sofa-surfing will not give you your desired outcome, for example.

Most importantly, however, is believing that you can do all of this. Believing in yourself, and not giving into the temptation to give up, is truly more important than anything else.

Having the conviction to eat a salad instead of cinnamon bun, or go for a jog instead of sitting on the sofa all night – that is what is important. And it is important to be proud of yourself every time you make a good choice. There will always be someone out there who is trying to drag you down –

even if it's your own inner thoughts – and if you want to succeed, you cannot let them hold you back.

Things that can help reverse type 2 diabetes:
- Increase activity level
- Lose weight
- Modify eating habits
- Fresh fruit and vegetables
- Whole grains
- Beans, legumes, nuts and seeds
- Wild-caught fatty fish, pasture-raised meats and poultry
- Chromium
- Vitamin D
- Vitamin C
- Beta-carotene
- Magnesium
- Probiotics
- Cinnamon
- Spirulina
- Chlorella
- Aloe vera
- Green tea
- Ginger
- Turmeric
- Astaxanthin
- Fish oil
- Whey protein
- Chia seeds
- Silymarin
- Selenium

And of course, believing in yourself is key!

References

1. "Type 2 Diabetes: MedlinePlus Medical Encyclopedia."
   U.S. National Library of Medicine.
   https://www.nlm.nih.gov/medlineplus/ency/article/000313.htm
   Retrieved: 1/12/16

2. "Overview - Type 2 diabetes." Mayo Clinic.
   http://www.mayoclinic.org/diseases-conditions/type-2-diabetes/home/ovc-20169860
   Retrieved: 3/16/16

3. "Symptoms and causes - Type 2 diabetes." Mayco Clinic.
   http://www.mayoclinic.org/diseases-conditions/type-2-diabetes/symptoms-causes/dxc-20169861
   Retrieved: 3/16/16

4. "Your Guide to Diabetes: Type 1 and Type 2." National Institute of Diabetes and Digestive and Kidney Diseases.
   http://www.niddk.nih.gov/health-information/health-topics/Diabetes/your-guide-diabetes/Pages/index.aspx
   Retrieved: 1/13/16

5. "Alzheimer's Disease Is Type-3 Diabetes—Evidence Reviewed." *Journal of Diabetes Science and Technology*.
   http://www.ncbi.nlm.nih.gov/pmc/articles/PMC2769828/
   Retrieved: 1/13/16

6. "Insulin Function, Insulin Resistance, and Food Intake Control of Secretion." *The Medical Biochemistry Page*.
   http://themedicalbiochemistrypage.org/insulin.php
   Retrieved: 1/14/16

7. "Signaling pathways in insulin action: molecular targets of insulin resistance." *The Journal of Clinical Investigation*.
   http://www.ncbi.nlm.nih.gov/pmc/articles/PMC314316/
   Retrieved: 1/12/16

8. Type 2 diabetes? It's 'walking deficiency syndrome' and not a real illness, says top doctor
   http://www.dailymail.co.uk/health/article-4362126/Type-2-diabetes-not-real-illness-says-doctor.html Retrieved: 4/13/17

9. "Insulin Resistance and Prediabetes." National Institute of Diabetes and Digestive and Kidney Diseases.
http://www.niddk.nih.gov/health-information/health-topics/Diabetes/insulin-resistance-pre-diabetes/Pages/index.aspx#happens
Retrieved: 1/13/16

10. "Poor control of diabetes may be linked to low vitamin D." Endocrine Society.
http://www.endocrine.org/news-room/press-release-archives/2010/poorcontrolofdiabetes-maybelinkedtolowvitamind
Retrieved: 1/13/16

11. "Glycemic index, glycemic load and risk of diabetes." *The American Journal of Clinical Nutrition*.
http://ajcn.nutrition.org/content/76/1/274S.long
Retrieved: 1/13/16

12. "Diabetes: Does alcohol and tobacco use increase my risk?" Mayo Clinic.
http://www.mayoclinic.org/diseases-conditions/type-2-diabetes/expert-answers/diabetes/faq-20058540
Retrieved: 1/13/16

13. "Symptoms and causes - Type 2 diabetes." Mayo Clinic.
http://www.mayoclinic.org/diseases-conditions/type-2-diabetes/symptoms-causes/dxc-20169861
Retrieved: 1/13/16

14. "What Causes Diabetic Heart Disease?" National Heart, Lung, and Blood Institute.
https://www.nhlbi.nih.gov/health/health-topics/topics/dhd/causes
Retrieved: 1/13/16

15. "Kidney Disease of Diabetes." National Institute of Diabetes and Digestive and Kidney Disease.
http://www.niddk.nih.gov/health-information/health-topics/kidney-disease/kidney-disease-of-diabetes/Pages/facts.aspx
Retrieved: 1/13/16

16. "Kidney Disease (Nephropathy)." American Diabetes Association.
http://www.diabetes.org/living-with-diabetes/complications/kidney-disease-nephropathy.html
Retrieved: 1/13/16

17. "Diabetes and Alzheimer's linked." Mayo Clinic.
http://www.mayoclinic.org/diabetes-and-alzheimers/art-20046987
Retrieved: 1/14/16

18. "Glycogen Synthesis and Metabolism." *The Medical Biochemistry Page*.
http://themedicalbiochemistrypage.org/glycogen.php
Retrieved: 1/14/16

19. "Diagnosis - Type 2 diabetes." Mayo Clinic.
http://www.mayoclinic.org/diseases-conditions/type-2-diabetes/diagnosis-treatment/diagnosis/dxc-20169894
Retrieved: 1/14/16

20. "Annual Number (in Thousands) of New Cases of Diagnosed Diabetes Among Adults Aged 18-79 Years, United States, 1980-2014." Centers for Disease Control and Prevention.
http://www.cdc.gov/diabetes/statistics/incidence/fig1.htm
Retrieved: 1/14/16

21. "Study: Diabetes increases years with disability, reduces lifespan." United Press International.
http://www.upi.com/Health_News/2016/01/06/Study-Diabetes-increases-years-with-disability-reduces-lifespan/4871452091449/
Retrieved: 1/14/16

22. "Childhood Obesity Facts." Centers for Disease Control and Prevention.
http://www.cdc.gov/healthyschools/obesity/facts.htm
Retrieved: 1/14/16

23. "Type 2 Diabetes in Youth: Epidemiology and Pathophysiology." *Diabetes Care*.
http://care.diabetesjournals.org/content/34/Supplement_2/S161.full
Retrieved: 1/14/16

24. "Number (in Millions) of Adults with Diabetes by Diabetes Medication Status, United States, 1997-2011." Centers for Disease Control and Prevention.
http://www.cdc.gov/diabetes/statistics/meduse/fig1.htm
Retrieved: 1/15/16

25. "For Patients Receiving Metformin to Treat Diabetes, Addition of Insulin Associated With Increased Risk of Death." The JAMA Network.
http://media.jamanetwork.com/news-item/for-patients-receiving-metformin-to-treat-diabetes-addition-of-insulin-associated-with-increased-risk-of-death/
Retrieved: 1/15/16

26. "What Are My Options?" American Diabetes Association.
http://www.diabetes.org/living-with-diabetes/treatment-and-care/medication/oral-medications/what-are-my-options.html
Retrieved: 1/15/16

27. "Initiating and Titrating Insulin in Patients with Type 2 Diabetes." *Clinical Diabetes*.
http://clinical.diabetesjournals.org/content/27/2/72.full
Retrieved: 1/15/16

28. "Dietary Guidelines After Bariatric Surgery." UCSF Medical Center.
http://www.ucsfhealth.org/education/dietary_guidelines_after_gastric_bypass/
Retrieved: 1/15/16

29. "Non-adherence in type 2 diabetes: practical considerations for interpreting the literature." *Patient Preference and Adherence*.
http://www.ncbi.nlm.nih.gov/pmc/articles/PMC3592508/
Retrieved: 1/15/16

30. "Why Treatment Fails in Type 2 Diabetes." *PLOS Medicine*.
http://journals.plos.org/plosmedicine/article?id=10.1371/journal.pmed.0050215
Retrieved: 1/18/16

31. "Insulin, Leptin, and Blood Sugar – Why Diabetic Medication Fails." Wellness Resources.
http://www.wellnessresources.com/health/articles/insulin_leptin_and_blood_sugar_why_diabetic_medication_fails/
Retrieved: 1/15/16

32. "What I need to know about Carbohydrate Counting and Diabetes." National Institute of Diabetes and Digestive and Kidney Diseases.
http://www.niddk.nih.gov/health-information/health-topics/Diabetes/carbohydrate-counting-diabetes/Pages/index.aspx
Retrieved: 1/18/16

33. "About Glycemic Index." GlycemicIndex.com.
http://www.glycemicindex.com/about.php
Retrieved: 1/18/16

34. "Doctors: 'Type 2 Diabetes Can Be Reversed!'" Death to Diabetes.
http://www.deathtodiabetes.com/Diabetes_Can_Be_Reversed.html#.Vp5a2LS4lo4
Retrieved: 1/19/16

35. "Why A Natural Approach To Treating Type 2 Diabetes Beats Medicine" *Mindbodygreen*.
http://www.mindbodygreen.com/0-8178/why-a-natural-approach-to-treating-type-2-diabetes-beats-medicine.html
Retrieved: 1/19/16

36. "Does Obesity Negate the Effects of Aerobic Exercise? Why These Experts Dismiss The 'Fat But Fit' Mentality." *Medical Daily*.
http://www.medicaldaily.com/does-obesity-negate-benefits-aerobic-exercise-why-these-experts-dismiss-fat-fit-366132
Retrieved: 1/19/16

37. "How to control type 2 diabetes in three steps." *Natural News*.
http://www.naturalnews.com/031638_type-2_diabetes_cure.html
Retrieved: 1/19/16

38. "Drastic lifestyle changes are best treatment for diabetes, obesity." *Natural News*
http://www.naturalnews.com/029918_diabetes_lifestyle_changes.html
Retrieved: 1/19/16

39. "Type 2 Diabetes: Etiology and reversibility." *Diabetes Care*.
http://care.diabetesjournals.org/content/36/4/1047.full
Retrieved: 1/19/16

40. "What Is Holistic Medicine?" *WebMD*.
http://www.webmd.com/balance/guide/what-is-holistic-medicine
Retrieved: 1/20/16

41. "Reversing Type 2 Diabetes With Natural Therapies." *Today's Dietitian*.
http://www.todaysdietitian.com/newarchives/111412p28.shtml
Retrieved: 1/20/16

42. "Macronutrients: the Importance of Carbohydrate, Protein and Fat." McKinley Health Center.
http://www.mckinley.illinois.edu/handouts/macronutrients.htm
Retrieved: 1/21/16

43. "Phytonutrients – Nature's Natural Defense." EatRight Ontario.
https://www.eatrightontario.ca/en/Articles/Antioxidants/Phytonutrients-–Nature's-Natural-Defense.aspx
Retrieved: 1/21/16

44. "Type 2 diabetes diet: What to eat, what to avoid and how to get healthier with every meal." *Natural News*.
http://www.naturalnews.com/045416_type_2_diabetes_diet_whole_grains.html
Retrieved: 1/21/16

45. "Carbohydrate Counting, Glycemic Index, and Glycemic Load: Putting Them All Together." *Diabetes Self-Management*.
http://www.diabetesselfmanagement.com/nutrition-exercise/meal-planning/carbohydrate-counting-glycemic-index-and-glycemic-load-putting-them-all-together/
Retrieved: 1/21/16

46. "Talking About *Trans* Fat: What You Need To Know." U.S. Food and Drug Administration.
http://www.fda.gov/Food/ResourcesForYou/Consumers/ucm079609.htm
Retrieved: 1/21/16

47. "Type 2 Diabetes Breakthrough: The Mediterranean Diet." *Natural News*.
http://www.naturalnews.com/027140_diet_diabetes_Type_2.html
Retrieved: 1/21/16

48. "The truth about low-fat foods." *BBC Good Food*.
http://www.bbcgoodfood.com/howto/guide/truth-about-low-fat-foods
Retrieved: 1/21/16

49. "Processed meat raises risk of diabetes, heart disease and cancer." *Natural News*.
http://www.naturalnews.com/028824_processed_meat_heart_disease.html
Retrieved: 1/21/16

50. "Studies show diet soda is linked to belly fat, type 2 diabetes and obesity." *Natural News*.
http://www.naturalnews.com/050123_diet_pop_soda_consumption_obesity.html
Retrieved: 1/21/16

51. "Artificial sweeteners may promote diabetes risk, but still promote weight loss." *Healthline*.

https://www.healthline.com/health-news/artificial-sweeteners-raise-diabetes-risk-091914
Retrieved: 1/21/16

52. "Soluble vs. insoluble fiber: MedlinePlus Medical Encyclopedia." U.S. National Library of Medicine.
https://www.nlm.nih.gov/medlineplus/ency/article/002136.htm
Retrieved: 1/22/16

53. "Whole Grains Found to Stabilize Blood Sugar For Up To Ten Hours." *Natural News*.
http://www.naturalnews.com/022490_grains_sugar_blood.html
Retrieved: 1/22/16

54. "Seafood – A Smart Choice for Diabetes." American Diabetes Association.
http://www.diabetes.org/mfa-recipes/tips/2012-08/seafood-a-smart-choice-for.html

55. "High Protein Diets Make People with Diabetes Manage Blood Sugar." *Medical Daily*.
http://www.medicaldaily.com/high-protein-foods-make-people-type-2-diabetes-manage-blood-sugar-353198
Retrieved: 1/22/16

56. "Role of Chromium in Human Health and in Diabetes." *Diabetes Care*.
http://care.diabetesjournals.org/content/27/11/2741.full
Retrieved: 1/22/16

57. "The Role of Vitamin D in Type 2 Diabetes." *Diabetes Forecast*.
http://www.diabetesforecast.org/2011/dec/the-role-of-vitamin-d-in-type-2-diabetes.html
Retrieved: 1/22/16

58. "The best dietary sources of vitamin D." *Natural News*.
http://www.naturalnews.com/047964_vitamin_D_dietary_sources_cod_liver_oil.html
Retrieved: 1/22/16

59. "12 Remarkable Untapped Potential and Healing Power of Vitamin C." *Natural News*.
http://blogs.naturalnews.com/12-remarkable-untapped-potential-healing-power-vitamin-c/
Retrieved: 1/25/16

60. "Diet High in Vitamin C Reduces Diabetes Risk." *Natural News*.
http://www.naturalnews.com/025605_vitamin_C_risk_diabetes.html
Retrieved: 1/25/16

61. "Top foods containing more vitamin C than an orange." *Natural News*.
http://www.naturalnews.com/045643_vitamin_C_oranges_healthy_foods.html
Retrieved: 1/25/16

62. "Beta carotene may protect from genetic Type II diabetes." *Natural News*.
http://www.naturalnews.com/038917_beta_carotene_type-2_diabetes_genetic_predisposition.html
Retrieved: 1/25/16

63. "The importance of beta carotene." *Natural News*.
http://www.naturalnews.com/037933_beta_carotene_carotenoids_foods.html
Retrieved: 1/25/16

64. "Magnesium in diet: MedlinePlus Medical Encyclopedia." U.S. National Library of Medicine.
https://www.nlm.nih.gov/medlineplus/ency/article/002423.htm
Retrieved: 1/25/16

65. "Magnesium Intake and Risk of Type 2 Diabetes in Men and Women." *Diabetes Care*.
http://care.diabetesjournals.org/content/27/1/134.full/Magnesium-Intake-and-Risk-of-Type-2-Diabetes-in-Men-and-Women
Retrieved: 1/25/16

66. "Top 10 magnesium-rich foods to boost your intake of this essential mineral." *Natural News*.
http://www.naturalnews.com/046094_magnesium-rich_foods_sources_essential_minerals.html
Retrieved: 1/25/16

67. "Sedentary lifestyle causes more deaths than smoking, says study." *Natural News*.
http://www.naturalnews.com/001547_sedentary_lifestyle_public_health.html
Retrieved: 1/26/16

68. "Young adults now only walk five minutes a day; Sedentary lifestyle the norm." *Natural News*.

http://www.naturalnews.com/042625_sedentary_lifestyle_young_adults_walking.html
Retrieved: 1/26/16

69. "Exercise in Itself Improves Blood Glucose Control in Type 2 Diabetes (press release)." *Natural News.*
http://www.naturalnews.com/020517_exercise_diabetes_blood.html
Retrieved: 1/26/16

70. "Research shows resistance exercise helps prevent type 2 diabetes." *Natural News.*
http://www.naturalnews.com/044348_type_2_diabetes_resistance_training_exercise.html
Retrieved: 1/26/16

71. "Smoking and Diabetes." Centers for Disease Control and Prevention.
http://www.cdc.gov/tobacco/campaign/tips/diseases/diabetes.html
Retrieved: 1/26/16

72. "Natural Diabetes Health: Ten Tips for Living with Type 2 Diabetes." *Natural News.*
http://www.naturalnews.com/025739_diabetes_blood_tips.html
Retrieved: 1/26/16

73. "Antidepressants again linked to type 2 diabetes risk." *Natural News.*
http://www.naturalnews.com/042396_antidepressants_type_2_diabetes_health_risks.html
Retrieved: 1/27/16

74. "Fast food diet increases risk of depression more than fifty percent." *Natural News.*
http://www.naturalnews.com/035772_fast_food_depression_nutrition.html
Retrieved: 1/27/16

75. "How to Conquer Depression Naturally." *Natural News.*
http://blogs.naturalnews.com/how-to-conquer-depression-naturally/
Retrieved: 1/27/16

76. Bacon, Linda. *Health at Every Size: The Surprising Truth about Your Weight.* Dallas, TX: BenBella, 2010. Print.

77. Obesity Paradox: Why Being Overweight May Not Matter as Much as You Think." *Natural News.*

http://blogs.naturalnews.com/obesity-paradox-overweight-might-not-matter-much-think/
Retrieved: 1/27/16

78. "Association of all-cause mortality with overweight and obesity using standard body mass index categories: a systematic review and meta-analysis." *The Journal of the American Medical Association*.
http://www.ncbi.nlm.nih.gov/pubmed/23280227
Retrieved: 1/27/16

79. Tribole, Evelyn; and Resch, Elyse. *Intuitive Eating: A Revolutionary Program That Works*. 3rd ed. New York: St. Martin's Griffin, 2012. Print.

80. "Probiotics are a MUST for type-2 diabetics: Research." *Natural News*.
http://www.naturalnews.com/041778_probiotics_type-2_diabetes_insulin_resistance.html
Retrieved: 1/28/16

81. "4 Probiotic Foods that Bulletproof the Immune System"
http://blogs.naturalnews.com/4-probiotic-foods-bulletproof-immune-system/
Retrieved: 1/28/16

82. "Cinnamon: the blood sugar stabilizer." *Natural News*.
http://www.naturalnews.com/035642_cinnamon_blood_sugar_regulating.html
Retrieved: 1/28/16

83. "Study touts spirulina as functional food for diabetes management." *Natural News*.
http://www.naturalnews.com/044455_spirulina_diabetes_management_functional_food.html
Retrieved: 1/29/16

84. "Studies show chlorella could improve insulin sensitivity in type 2 diabetes patients." *Natural News*.
http://www.naturalnews.com/042773_chlorella_insulin_sensitivity_type_2_diabetes.html
Retrieved: 1/29/16

85. "The aloe vera miracle: A natural medicine for cancer, cholesterol, diabetes, inflammation, IBS, and other health conditions." *Natural News*.
http://www.naturalnews.com/021858_aloe_vera_gel.html
Retrieved: 1/29/16

86. "Green tea extract may help prevent type-2 diabetes through improved glucose tolerance." *Natural News.*
http://www.naturalnews.com/020705_diabetes_prevention_EGCG.html
Retrieved: 1/29/16

87. "Green tea: a refreshing way to manage type 2 diabetes." *Natural News.*
http://blogs.naturalnews.com/green-tea-refreshing-way-manage-type-2-diabetes/
Retrieved: 1/29/16

88. "Ginger for type 2 diabetics: This power herb is scientifically proven to increase insulin sensitivity." *Natural News.*
http://www.naturalnews.com/040970_ginger_diabetes_insulin_resistance.html
Retrieved: 1/29/16

89. "Turmeric Shows Promise in Combating Diabetes and Obesity." *Natural News.*
http://www.naturalnews.com/024226_diabetes_turmeric_curcumin.html
Retrieved: 1/29/16

90. "Astaxanthin: The Little-Known Miracle Nutrient for Inflammation, Anti-Aging, Athletic Endurance and More." *Natural News.*
http://www.naturalnews.com/023177_astaxanthin_antioxidants.html
Retrieved: 2/1/16

91. "New science says fish oil prevents type 2 diabetes." *Natural News.*
http://www.naturalnews.com/040697_type_2_diabetes_omega-3_disease_prevention.html
Retrieved: 2/1/16

92. "Study proves omega-3 fatty acids lower risk of type 2 diabetes." *Natural News.*
http://www.naturalnews.com/043654_omega-3_fatty_acids_type_2_diabetes_disease_prevention.html
Retrieved: 2/1/16

93. "Whey protein lowers diabetes and cardiovascular disease risk factors in obese adults." *Natural News.*
http://www.naturalnews.com/045202_whey_protein_obesity_diabetes_prevention.html
Retrieved: 2/1/16

94. "Study shows milk thistle extract treats diabetes by lowering blood sugar, protecting liver." *Natural News.*

http://www.naturalnews.com/020971_milk_thistle_diabetes.html
Retrieved: 2/1/16

95. "Studies show that chia seeds can treat diabetes, boost energy and more." *Natural News*.
http://www.naturalnews.com/043250_chia_seeds_diabetes_treatment_essential_fatty_acids.html
Retrieved: 2/1/16

96. "Serum Selenium and Diabetes in U.S. Adults." *Diabetes Care*.
http://care.diabetesjournals.org/content/30/4/829.long
Retrieved: 2/1/16

97. "A Randomized Trial of Selenium Supplementation and Risk of Type-2 Diabetes, as Assessed by Plasma Adiponectin." *PLOS ONE*.
http://journals.plos.org/plosone/article?id=10.1371/journal.pone.0045269
Retrieved: 2/1/16

98. The best and worst forms of magnesium to take as a supplement
http://www.naturalnews.com/046401_magnesium_dietary_supplements_nutrient_absorption.html
Retrieved: 4/13/17

Notes: